Handbook

Sports Me

and Science

Road Cycling

D1645798

**Road cycling by Conconi,
Francesco**

IOC Medical Commission
Sub-commission on Publications
in the Sport Sciences

Howard G. Knuttgen PhD (Co-ordinator)
Boston, Massachusetts, USA

Francesco Conconi MD
Ferrara, Italy

Harm Kuipers MD, PhD
Maastricht, The Netherlands

Per A.F.H. Renström MD, PhD
Stockholm, Sweden

Richard H. Strauss MD
Los Angeles, California, USA

Handbook of
Sports Medicine
and Science
Road Cycling

EDITED BY

Robert J. Gregor

Department of Health & Performance Sciences
Georgia Institute of Technology
Atlanta
GA 30332–0110
USA

Francesco Conconi

Professor of Applied Biochemistry
University of Ferrara
Via Gramicia 35
I-44100 Ferrara
Italy

**Blackwell
Science**

© 2000
Blackwell Science Ltd
Editorial Offices:
Osney Mead, Oxford OX2 0EL
25 John Street, London WC1N 2BL
23 Ainslie Place, Edinburgh EH3 6AJ
350 Main Street, Malden
 MA 02148 5018, USA
54 University Street, Carlton
 Victoria 3053, Australia
10, rue Casimir Delavigne
 75006 Paris, France

Other Editorial Offices:
Blackwell Wissenschafts-Verlag GmbH
Kurfürstendamm 57
10707 Berlin, Germany

Blackwell Science KK
MG Kodenmacho Building
7–10 Kodenmacho Nihombashi
Chuo-ku, Tokyo 104, Japan

First published 2000

Set by Graphicraft Limited, Hong Kong
Printed and bound in Great Britain by
MPG Books Ltd, Bodmin, Cornwall

The Blackwell Science logo is a
trade mark of Blackwell Science Ltd,
registered at the United Kingdom
Trade Marks Registry

A catalogue record for this title
is available from the British Library

ISBN 0–86542–912–X

Library of Congress
Cataloging-in-publication Data
Road cycling/edited by Robert J. Gregor,
 Francesco Conconi.
   p. ; cm. (Handbook of sports
 medicine and science)
 Includes index.
 ISBN 0-86542-912-X
 1. Cycling—Physiological aspects.
2. Sports medicine. 3. Biomechanics.
I. Gregor, Robert J. II. Conconi,
Francesco, 1935– . III. Series.
[DNLM: 1. Bicycling—physiology.
2. Biomechanics. 3. Sports Medicine.
QT 260.5.B5 R628 2000]
RC1220.C8 R63 2000
612′.044—dc21

                99–046476

DISTRIBUTORS
Marston Book Services Ltd
PO Box 269
Abingdon, Oxon OX14 4YN
(Orders: Tel: 01235 465500
        Fax: 01235 465555)

USA
Blackwell Science, Inc.
Commerce Place
350 Main Street
Malden, MA 02148 5018
(Orders: Tel: 800 759 6102
           781 388 8250
        Fax: 781 388 8255)

Canada
Login Brothers Book Company
324 Saulteaux Crescent
Winnipeg, Manitoba R3J 3T2
(Orders: Tel: 204 837 2987)

Australia
Blackwell Science Pty Ltd
54 University Street
Carlton, Victoria 3053
(Orders: Tel: 3 9347 0300
        Fax: 3 9347 5001)

For further information on
Blackwell Science, visit our website:
www.blackwell-science.com

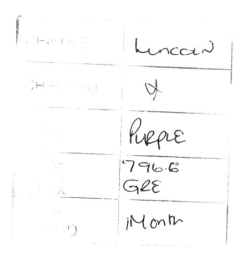

Contents

List of contributors

Nicola Alfieri MD, *Centro Studi Biomedici Applicati allo Sport, Università degli Studi di Ferrara, Via Gramicia 35, I-44100 Ferrara, Italia*

Arnold Baker MD, CM, CCFP, ABFP, *1820 Washington Place, San Diego, CA 92103, USA*

Frederick Brouns MD, *Sibberkerkstraat 38, NL-6301 AW Valkenburg, The Netherlands*

Jeffrey P. Broker PhD, *Sport Science and Technology Division, United States Olympic Training Center, 1 Olympic Plaza, Colorado Springs, CO 80909, USA*

Francesco Conconi MD, *Professor of Applied Biochemistry, Università degli Studi di Ferrara, Via Gramicia 35, I-44100 Ferrara, Italia*

Robert J. Gregor PhD, *Professor and Head of Department, Department of Health & Performance Sciences, Georgia Institute of Technology, Atlanta, GA 30332–0110, USA*

Forewords

A sustained interest in improving competitive performance has resulted in biomechanical research that has provided innovative changes in the design of both the bicycle and the athlete's attire. Physiological research has changed the conditioning programmes and nutritional strategies. This publication will benefit all scientific, medical and coaching personnel who work with competitive cyclists.

PRINCE ALEXANDRE DE MERODE
Chairman, IOC Medical Commission

On behalf of the International Olympic Committee I should like to welcome the new volume in our Handbook of Sports Medicine series, *Road Cycling*, published in this very important year, the year of the Games of XXVII Olympiad to be celebrated in Sydney.

This text brings together expertise from France, Holland, Italy and the United States to present an authoritative reference on training techniques and medical problems encountered in competitive cycling.

My sincere thanks go to Prince Alexandre de Merode and the Publications in Sport Sciences sub-commission of the IOC Medical Commission.

JUAN ANTONIO SAMARANCH
Marqués de Samaranch

On behalf of the International Olympic Committee and its Medical Commission, I should like to welcome this important publication written by an eminent group of authorities from basic, applied and clinical science, representing the latest information on the biomechanics, physiology, nutrition and medical aspects of cycling.

Cycling is one of the toughest sports and one of the most complex to analyse in scientific terms.

Numerous technical and medical factors form the basis of the extraordinary relationship, which, for more than a century, has connected people with the bicycle. All those who cycle, whether cycle-tourists or great champions, need to have detailed knowledge about the discipline they have chosen.

This book is thus extremely valuable and contains all the necessary facts and information that all cyclists need in order to fully appreciate their love of cycling.

The skill with which the authors present the subject provides us with an excellent source of reference which will be useful to millions and gives an ideal approach on the most sensitive of subjects, such as training and diet.

The International Cycling Union (UCI) is therefore pleased to be associated with the publication of a book which will make a significant contribution to developing the culture of cycling.

HEIN VERBRUGGEN
President, UCI

Acknowledgements

We would first like to thank the International Olympic Committee, its Medical Commission, Prince Alexandre de Merode, and specifically the Publication's Advisory Committee for their foresight in the development of these handbooks. We recognize that the Medical Commission will continue to devote substantial effort and enthusiasm to the cause of scientific research as it relates to human movement and physical activity in sport. We feel this Handbook on Road Cycling will contribute to this cause and to the improvement of cyclists around the world. We would also like to recognize the tireless efforts and contributions made by Howard G. Knuttgen. He has toiled long and well for this project and has seen it to fruition. Finally, we would like to thank the International Cycling Federation for their support of this handbook. We feel it will make a substantial contribution to cycling science and that the objective of practical application of scientific information to the world of sport is realized in this handbook.

As editors, we wish to acknowledge the valuable contributions to the production of this handbook of each of the contributing authors listed in the table of contents. These authors either completely wrote or significantly contributed to the chapters cited following their names. This was truly an international effort.

Chapter 1

Anatomy, biochemistry and physiology of road cycling

Skeletal muscle anatomy

Skeletal muscle is a transformer designed to convert signals from the nervous system and chemical energy from food substrates into force to produce and control movement. While muscle fibres possess certain physiological characteristics, they are joined to the bone through a tendon. Some properties of muscle are described with respect to the fibres themselves, but more realistically, the performance of muscle must be considered in light of its interaction with the tendon and, subsequently, the bone. It is this muscle–tendon unit which deals with the real world and possesses certain mechanical properties, controlled by impulses from sensory and motor portions of the nervous system, that performs the different functions in movement control.

The discussion in this chapter is devoted to the mechanical properties of skeletal muscle and the application of our understanding of these properties to normal movements. Discussion will focus on (i) muscle architecture, (ii) muscle fibre length, (iii) physiological cross-sectional area, (iv) the motor unit and (v) how compartments within muscle are used as synergists.

Basic architecture of the muscle begins with the sarcomere as the structural unit of skeletal muscle fibres. This repeating unit represents the region of the myofibril from one Z line to another and essentially is an area of interdigitating myofilaments (Fig. 1.1). At rest, the sarcomere is approximately 2.0–2.25 μm in length. Each myofibril is composed of bundles of myofilaments and the obvious striations in skeletal muscle are due to the differential refraction of light as it passes through the contractile proteins in these filaments. The thick and thin filaments, and the different proteins found within each filament, are considered to be the fundamental elements controlling force and contraction velocity. The thinner filament structure is dominated by the actin molecule (Fig. 1.2). The major role of this actin filament is interaction with the myosin filament. The main constituent of the thick filament is the protein myosin, which is a larger molecule than actin (Fig. 1.2). The myosin filament contains the cross-bridges which are identical protein heads that, in the proper circumstances, connect to the actin filament. It is this bonding to the actin filament that results in the generation of force. Once these conditions are achieved, these two proteins bind together, the heads rotate and the muscle contracts towards the centre of the sarcomere. This contraction towards the centre then propagates down the muscle fibre, resulting in fibre shortening and, subsequently, shortening of the whole muscle.

Sarcomeres are arranged in series to form a skeletal muscle fibre. The longer the fibre, the greater the number of sarcomeres in series and the faster the shortening velocity of that fibre. The relationship between fibre length and maximum shortening velocity has been described in the scientific literature for many years.

An additional feature of muscle architecture, aside from the repeating sarcomeres in series creating fibres of different lengths, is the fact that fibres are arranged at certain angles from the long axis of the muscle. Some muscles have greater angles of pinnation than others, with some fibres at angles approximating 40°. Other muscles have fibres that might be only 3 or 4° from the long axis of the muscle. Since fibres are arranged at different angles of pinnation, we have unipinnate, paralleled fibred and multipinnate muscles, all of which represent the range of organization of muscle fibres with respect to the pulling axis of the muscle. The different angles of pinnation also result in different physiological cross-sectional areas of separate muscles. The greater the angle of pinnation, the greater the physiological cross-sectional area (PCSA) that the muscle contains. The greater the area, typically the more protein and typically the higher amount of force produced by that muscle.

What has been presented thus far is information related to the speed of muscle contraction, related to its fibre length and the magnitude of force that a muscle might produce, as related to its PCSA. Consequently, by design, muscles are organized in ways

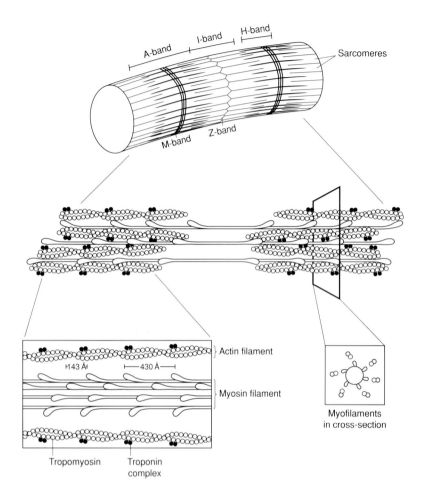

Fig. 1.1 Hexagonal array of interdigitating actin and myosin filaments (myofilaments), which comprise the sarcomere. Arranged at intervals along the actin filament are the regulatory proteins troponin and tropomyosin. Reproduced with permission from Lieber (1992).

that make them either faster, by virtue of fibre length, or stronger and capable of higher forces, by virtue of their angle of pinnation and its effect on PCSA.

In addition to its fibre length, the speed of muscle contraction is controlled by the form of myosin contained in the myosin filaments which is the thick filament, described above. The myosin filament, which contains the cross-bridges capable of connecting to actin, has different forms. These forms describe our muscles as fast or slow. In other words, if we have fast myosin, the heads on the cross-bridges will rotate rapidly. If the myosin form is slow, then our muscles are primarily considered to be slow-twitch muscles, and the heads of the myosin filaments will rotate slowly. The metabolic functions of these two types of myosin are also quite different but, in short, if we have a fast type of myosin we are considered to have fast-twitch fibres, and if we have a slow type of myosin, we

are considered to have slow-twitch fibres. In the literature, scientists have presented 55 different forms of myosin yielding a virtual continuum of speed capabilities on the part of the muscle. Athletes are usually characterized according to slow-twitch or fast-twitch muscles and those categories are rather distinct. However, it must be remembered that we really have a much broader spectrum of myosin types, leading to a variety of speed capabilities within skeletal muscle.

Two general properties of muscle, commonly referred to as physiological properties of muscle, are the length–tension curve (Fig. 1.3) and the force–velocity curve (Fig. 1.4). In Fig. 1.3(a), we see the active length–tension curve. This essentially tells us that cross-bridges overlap in some optimal way and, if the muscle is activated while they are in that position, maximum tension will be generated. As the muscle

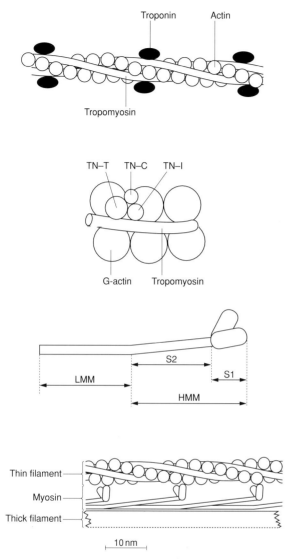

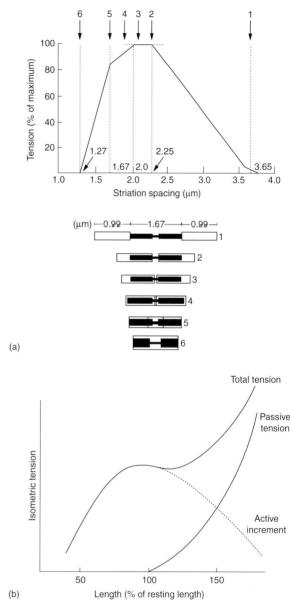

Fig. 1.2 The troponin and tropomyosin molecules on the actin filament together with subfragments of the troponin molecule (TN–T = troponin–T; TN–I = troponin–I; TN–C = tropon in–C). In addition, the structure of the myocin thick filament showing light meromyosin (LMM) and heavy meromyosin (HMM) with subfragments S2 and S1 is shown. The S1 fragment is the globular head of the cross-bridge that links to the actin filament during muscle contraction.

Fig. 1.3 (a) The active length–tension curve of an isolated sarcomere, showing the effect of filament overlap on tension generation under maximal stimulation. (b) Active length–tension curve together with the passive length–tension curve. The summation of these two curves represents the total tension curve. Passive tension comes primarily from the tendon and other protein structures within the muscle that produce tension in a lengthening contraction with no stimulation by the nervous system.

shortens tension will decrease and as muscle lengthens tension will also reduce because the filaments will not be in an ideal position to generate force. The centre of the length–tension curve is the optimal overlap of the cross-bridges and, as the interdigitating

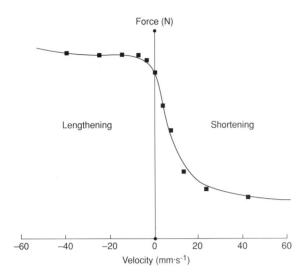

Fig. 1.4 The force–velocity curve for skeletal muscle during both shortening and lengthening contractions. Zero velocity represents maximum isometric contraction: increases in shortening velocity show exponential decreases in tension and increases in lengthening velocity show exponential increases. Ultimately tension production reaches a plateau.

filaments come closer together, tension declines; as they are pulled further apart, tension will reduce despite the amount of activation received from the nervous system.

The passive length–tension curve is presented in Fig. 1.3(b). The passive length–tension curve shows an increase in tension as the muscle is stretched beyond its resting length. If the muscle receives no activation from the nervous system and is stretched, it will resist the stretching force, yielding a force output on the part of that whole muscle–tendon unit. Finally, if we combine the active portion of the length–tension curve, i.e. when the muscle receives maximal excitation from the nervous system, and the passive length–tension curve, we see what is referred to as the total tension curve, which is a combination of both the active and passive components (Fig. 1.3b). This information tells us that muscle length is a primary requisite to tension development, whether the muscle is activated by the nervous system or not.

On the force–velocity curve, presented in Fig. 1.4, we see a portion that begins at a very high force, commonly referred to as maximal isometric tension, when the muscle is neither shortening nor lengthening. As we proceed to the positive side, or the shortening

velocity side of the force–velocity curve, we see that, as speed increases, force reduces. The theoretical point at maximum velocity yields no force production capabilities by the muscle. This point is outside the normal range that individuals experience in normal movements. In normal movements, there is never a situation where muscle is contracting so fast that it is incapable of producing force.

The interesting part of the force–velocity curve lies in the lengthening contraction of the muscle (Fig. 1.4). We see an increase in force and then a plateau in force production capabilities as the velocity of lengthening increases. This is an important part of the force–velocity curve since, in most normal movements, lengthening contractions precede shortening contractions. Specifically, in cycling the quadriceps muscles responsible for extending the knee are first lengthening as the leg comes up to top dead centre in crank position, and then shorten as the rider extends the knee during the power phase. This is an important point to remember because muscles in the legs always lengthen before shortening during force production to turn the crank. Finally, the profile of the length–tension curve can be affected by the geometry of the muscle. For example, the plateau of maximum force capability will be extended to a wider range if the fibre is long. Also, the force–velocity curve is affected by the type of myosin. Slow-twitch myosin results in lower force and lower maximum velocity capabilities, while fast-twitch myosin has higher force and higher maximum velocities of contraction. All these factors are closely related and will affect the ultimate force production capabilities of the muscle in dynamic situations such as cycling.

So far, we have discussed the fundamental structural components of skeletal muscle in relation to sarcomeres in series yielding long fibres, PCSA of the muscle in relation to muscle force production capabilities, and biochemistry in relation to the functions of the actin and myosin filaments and the speed of the muscle contraction. While we consider these elements fundamental structural units of muscle, the functional unit of skeletal muscle is typically referred to as the motor unit (Fig. 1.5). A motor unit consists of a single motor axon innervating a number of skeletal muscle fibres. One motor unit with a single motor axon may contain only four fibres, e.g. ocular muscles, and up to several hundred fibres in the large muscles of the leg

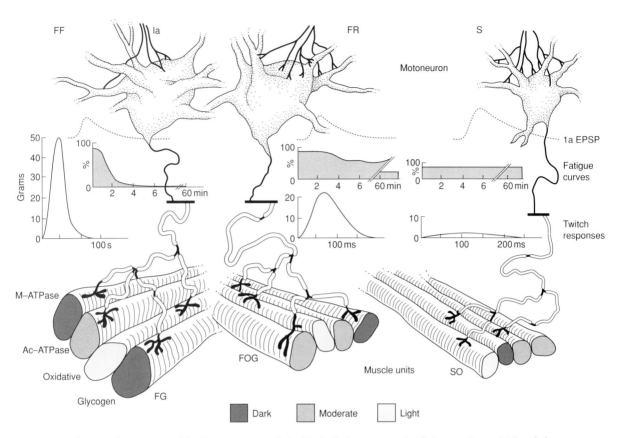

Fig. 1.5 Fundamental properties of the fast-contracting fatigable (FF), fast-contracting fatigue-resistant (FR) and slow-contracting fatigue-resistant (S) motor units in relation to recruitment order, tension development, fatigue resistance, myosin adenosine triphosphatase activity, oxidative capacity and glycogen content. FG, fast glycolytic; FOG, fast oxidative glycolytic; SO, slow oxidative; 1a, a nerve; EPSP, excitatory post-synaptic potential. Reproduced with permission from Burke and Edgerton (1975).

and back. The fibres in each motor unit contract simultaneously once the motor nerve excites the muscle fibres as a unit. The more fibres we have and the larger they are, the greater the tension production capabilities. The fewer fibres in a motor unit, and the smaller they are, the smaller the tension production.

A motor unit is generally considered to be all fast or all slow. Whatever myosin type exists within the muscle fibre, it is considered to be generally the same motor unit. Hence, we have slow motor units recruited by the nervous system and fast motor units recruited by the nervous system. If we consider a situation where muscle is required to produce gradual increases in force in an isometric contraction, the nervous system will first recruit the slow, smaller, lower

tension production motor units and then proceed through the continuum until it activates the faster, larger-fibred greater tension production capability motor units. This feature of the neural control of muscle is generally referred to as the size principle.

Motor axons innervating slow motor units have small cell bodies and are depolarized first, while motor axons innervating large fast fibres in a fast motor unit have a large cell body and are depolarized last (Fig. 1.5). The two principles governing how motor units produce tension and subsequently how the muscle produces force focus on, firstly, the recruitment of motor units, and secondly, the firing frequency of those motor units. In a sense, we recruit a motor unit to produce a certain amount of tension and, if

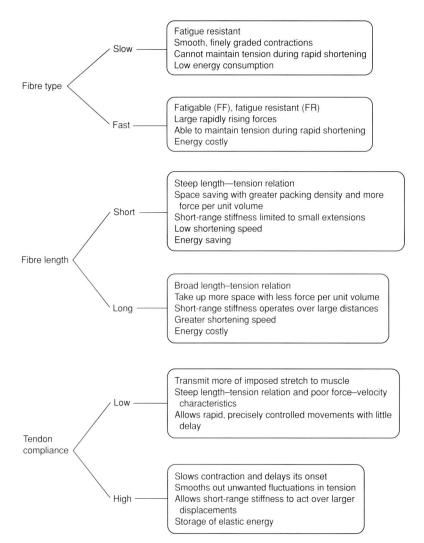

Fig. 1.6 Relationship between major factors influencing the performance of the muscle tendon unit in movement control. Reproduced with permission from Walmsley and Proske (1981).

tension is increased, more motor units are recruited. Once a motor unit is activated by the nervous system, the only other option to increase force in that motor unit is to increase its firing rate. Recruitment is a major feature of muscle force increase and rate coding (increasing tension by virtue of increasing the rate of firing) is a secondary way the nervous system can increase force production capabilities in a selected muscle.

Finally, to enhance our understanding of how these different properties of muscle are coordinated during normal movement, we refer to Fig. 1.6. This figure shows the properties of two types of motor units, slow and fast, two general types of fibre length, short and

long, and two types of tendon compliance, low and high. Coordinating the various features of the muscle tendon unit then becomes a complicated process. For example, we could have a fast muscle with short fibres capable of producing a great deal of force in a short period of time connected to a relatively long tendon. The fact that the tendon is long and compliant means that the force produced by those muscle fibres will not reach the bone quickly because the first responsibility of the contracting fibres is to take up the compliance, or slack, in the tendon. Another extreme situation might be a slow fibre with a long fibre length and a short tendon. The tension produced in the fibres would be lower than in fast fibres, while the length of the fibre will affect the speed of contraction and the length–tension curve. The fact that we have a short tendon also means that whatever tension is developed will reach the bone in a relatively short period of time. By design, the musculoskeletal system has muscles of different cross-sectional areas, fibre lengths, fibre types and tendon lengths, leaving us with a variety of resources capable of controlling movement in selected ways when activated by the nervous system.

We should now have an understanding of the design of the muscular system and the breadth of resources available to the nervous system in its con-trol of movement. When activated by the nervous system, muscle fibres will produce force and shorten unless acted upon by an external force. This activation process changes the mechanical properties of the muscle and modulates the physiological properties of the muscle as it interfaces with the mechanical tendon. The resources available to the nervous system are important when learning a task in controlling movement. For further information on these muscle properties, see the large number of textbooks on muscle physiology available in the literature.

Muscle activity patterns during cycling (Fig. 1.7)

The information presented here relates to the muscle activity patterns of 10 major muscles in the legs. The literature has very little information on muscles in the back, neck or upper extremities, and a great deal of information on patterns of activity of major hip, knee and ankle flexors and extensors. While the upper extremities and back are important to cycling and should not be discounted in training, most available information on how muscles function during cycling describe the major leg muscles.

Figure 1.8 shows the average activity patterns from a position in the pedalling cycle between 0°, when the crank is at top dead centre (TDC), and 360°, when the crank has returned to its vertical upright position. The point 180° in crank rotation represents the position when the crank is vertically down at the bottom dead centre portion of the pedalling cycle. The range of motion from 0 to 180° is considered to be the power phase of cycling and from 180 to 360° is the recovery phase. Muscles active in the power phase produce force against the crank in an effort to rotate the crank. Muscle activity observed during recovery may have several functions:

1 producing enough activity and force to lift the leg;
2 producing a small amount of activity, resulting in inadequate force production, leaving the leg to rest on the crank and forcing the other leg to push harder;
3 producing a great deal of activity and force to lift and help rotate the crank to power the bike.

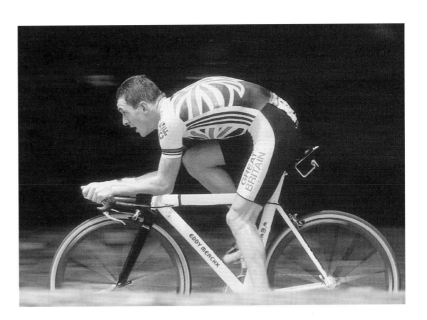

Fig. 1.7 Atlanta 1996: individual time trial. Chris Boardman (GBR) using muscle patterns shown in Fig. 1.8, third. © Allsport / Pascal Rondeau.

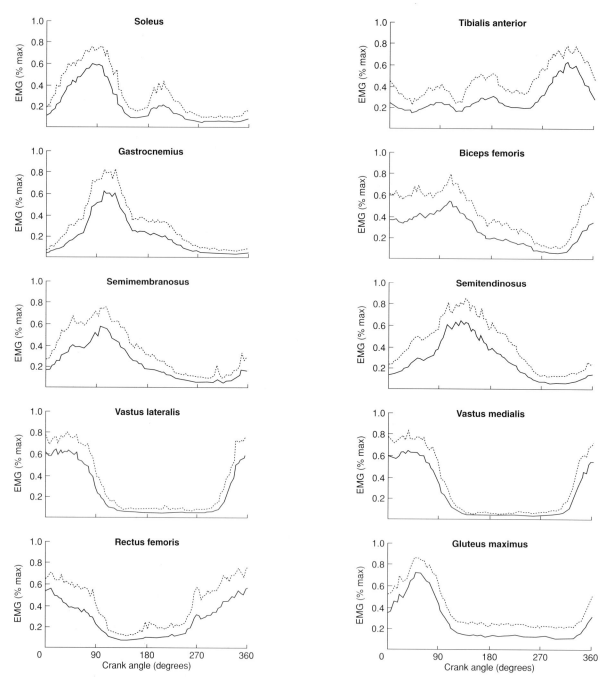

Fig. 1.8 Average patterns of muscle activation during the pedalling cycle for 10 muscles in the human lower extremity. The solid line is the average pattern of 15 pedalling cycles across 18 subjects (270 cycles) and the dashed curve is 1 s.d. above the mean. Magnitudes are normalized to maximal activation. Reproduced with permission from Ryan and Gregor (1992).

In any event, if a muscle is active and shows much activity, it is important to the nervous system and to the control of crank rotation during cycling.

Representative data from 18 experienced cyclists riding their own racing bicycles at 90 rpm and 250 W are shown in Fig. 1.8. During the propulsive phase, power is imparted to the bike through forceful hip and knee extension. The gluteus maximus and quadriceps muscles are heavily recruited during this time. For example, onset of activity for the gluteus maximus occurs just before TDC; peak activity is observed just after TDC at approximately 55° of crank rotation. Both medial and lateral vasti muscles, which are single-joint knee extensors, exhibit a rapid onset and cessation with relatively constant activity in between. The rectus femoris, on the other hand, which is a hip flexor and knee extensor, demonstrates a more gradual rise and decline. Rectus femoris activity onset occurs before the vasti muscles and declines earlier in the power phase. This is most likely to be due to its additional function as a hip extensor. Electromyogram (EMG) readings show a drop shortly after 90° of crank rotation, when all three muscles end their role as significant contributors to the work necessary to drive the bicycle.

Major ankle extensors are also active during the propulsive phase and, while not considered major power producers, are important in providing a stable link between the pedal, the foot, and the more proximal joints, hip and knee. These ankle extensors ensure that the total amount of energy produced in lower-extremity musculature can be transmitted to the pedal. The soleus, a single-joint ankle extensor, is recruited just before the gastrocnemius, an ankle extensor and knee flexor, and both muscles are active before TDC, with peak activity occurring before 90° in the pedalling cycle. The gastrocnemius is recruited shortly after the soleus and peak activity occurs at an average of 107° after TDC, declining gradually during recovery and ending at approximately 270° of crank rotation. This phase shift in soleus relative to gastrocnemius onset may be related to two factors: firstly, peak stretch occurs later in the gastrocnemius than the soleus (see data presented in Chapter 2) and in both muscles peak EMG seems to occur just before peak stretch, and secondly, a delayed peak in the activation of the gastrocnemius contributes to a knee flexor moment consistently observed after 90° in the

pedal cycle (see Chapter 2). Force enhancement may occur in these muscles due to the presence of active stretch before muscle shortening for both the gastrocnemius and soleus muscles. Additionally, the tibialis anterior, a single-joint ankle flexor, is active during the propulsive phase in many individuals. When observed, it is coactive with the ankle extensors and may be used to enhance ankle stability during propulsion and force transmission to the pedal.

The hamstring muscles are also active during the power phase of cycling functioning, in part as hip extensors. The semimembranosus and semitendinosus are recruited after TDC and peak activity occurs at, or slightly after, 90° when activity in the gluteal and vasti muscles is rapidly declining. Peak activity in the semitendinosus occurs slightly after that of the semimembranosus, and biceps femoris activity is the most variable of all three hamstrings. In some individuals, timing of the biceps femoris is similar to the semimembranosus and semitendinosus while in others it is already maximally active at TDC and declines throughout propulsion. Finally, continued activation of the hamstrings for the remainder of the power phase contributes to the knee flexor moment, especially in the absence of any quadriceps activity after 90° of crank rotation. As stated above, joint kinetic data will be presented in detail in Chapter 2.

During the recovery phase, from 180 to 360° in the pedalling cycle, the lower extremity flexes and serves two functions: firstly, it reduces the resistance on the crank to the propulsive phase on the contralateral limb, and secondly, it provides enough flexion to rotate the crank and assist the contralateral limb in propulsion. Initially (between 180° and 235° of the pedalling cycle), the hamstrings and gastrocnemius muscles are active and provide a major component to flex the knee. Later in the recovery phase, between 235° and 360°, the tibialis anterior is active to dorsiflex the ankle. At the same time, the rectus femoris is active and can serve to flex the hip. Unfortunately, no information is available on the iliopsoas muscle, which is a single-joint hip flexor. As a result, it is unknown how active this muscle is. The fact remains, however, that the hip actively flexes during the recovery phase and, as a result, we assume that the iliopsoas is active during this portion of the pedalling cycle.

Almost all the data presented on EMG patterns in the lower extremity during cycling have been collected using surface electrodes. While good agreement has been found between surface electrodes and data from experiments using fine wire electrodes in the evaluation of large muscles, few studies are available on the results of using fine wire electrodes.

Finally while the patterns presented for the 10 major muscles are fairly robust and change very little, timing of the muscle activity patterns may be affected by seat height change, acceleration of the crank and possibly the position of the rider on the bicycle.

In summary, the major points regarding muscle activity during the cycling task are as follows.

1 Coactivation of knee flexors and extensors appears during the first 90° of the pedalling cycle while both the hamstring muscle group and the gastrocnemius muscle continue being active through the remainder of the power phase and during the recovery phase.

2 Single-joint muscle activity, e.g. the soleus muscle, is consistent across subjects, while activity patterns in biarticular multijoint muscles are much more variable.

3 Almost all the muscles in the lower extremity begin their activation pattern during muscle stretch and some of the activation ends before the muscle has completed its shortening phase.

Energy metabolism in cycling

Adenosine triphosphate and muscular contraction

To perform work, it is necessary to spend energy. Energy is available in different forms: in a battery, for example, as electrical energy, or in combustibles, as chemical energy. Chemical energy is energy stored in the bonds between atoms.

Cells contain adenosine triphosphate (ATP), a molecule composed of adenosine, to which three phosphate groups are attached (Fig. 1.9). ATP is essential to cellular activities, including muscular work; without ATP, muscular contraction is impossible. The chemical energy used for these activities is that stored in the bonds connecting the phosphate groups. When the second phosphate bond is broken, this bonding energy becomes available to

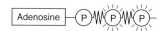

Fig. 1.9 Adenosine triphosphate (ATP).

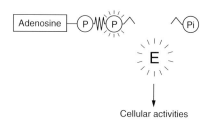

Fig. 1.10 The bonding energy is now available to the cell.

the cell (Fig. 1.10). The first phosphate bond can also be used on occasion.

Muscular availability of ATP

ATP is present in muscle fibres in a concentration of 2.5 g for every kilogram of tissue. Its total muscle availability is approximately 50 g. ATP molecules are quickly degraded to adenosine diphosphate (ADP). During maximal effort, such as a sprint, the available ATP is completely utilized and its muscle stores are completely exhausted in less than 1 s if adequate mechanisms of resynthesis do not function.

Resynthesis of ATP

ATP resynthesis from creatine phosphate (anaerobic alactacid resynthesis)

The fastest mechanism of ATP resynthesis uses the phosphate groups of creatine phosphate (CP) (Fig. 1.11). CP is composed of a molecule called creatine to which one phosphate group is attached. As soon as ATP begins to be degraded to ADP, a

Fig. 1.11 Creatine phosphate.

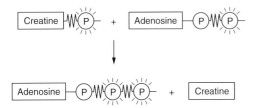

Fig. 1.12 Transfer of the phosphate group CP to ADP.

specific enzyme, called creatine kinase, activates the transfer of the phosphate group of CP to ADP. Since this transfer occurs rapidly, exhaustion of the ATP stores is prevented (Fig. 1.12). However, the CP stores are depleted.

CP is stored in a greater quantity than ATP: the number of CP molecules contained in the muscle cells is, on average, five times greater than that of ATP. The muscle CP concentration varies from subject to subject and is greater in sprinters and athletes from sports that require rapid acceleration than in endurance athletes.

ATP and CP are used simultaneously in brief intense efforts. Used together, the two molecules allow for a maximal effort lasting 4–8 s, depending on the individual's creatine concentration.

Under conditions of prolonged maximal effort, such as a long sprint or an attempt to close a gap in cycling, during which ATP and CP stores may be almost depleted, ADP may also be utilized and degraded to adenosine monophosphate (AMP). As a consequence of this reaction, ADP availability is also reduced, while AMP concentration increases. The excess AMP is used in a reaction that produces ammonia, a toxic byproduct, that accumulates in an athlete during a long sprint as well as in endurance competitions.

ATP resynthesis from breakdown of organic fuels

To sustain prolonged muscular activity, two additional mechanisms of ATP resynthesis are available: firstly, the aerobic mechanism, which is based on the breakdown of organic fuels with the use of oxygen (O_2), and secondly, the anaerobic mechanism, based on the partial breakdown of glucose without O_2.

Aerobic mechanism of ATP resynthesis

The O_2 necessary to sustain the aerobic mechanism reaches the muscle cells via respiration, absorption by the lungs, passage to the red blood cells, transport to the tissues via the cardiocirculatory system, and transfer from the red blood cells to the tissues, where it is utilized to 'burn' organic fuels, releasing the energy required for ATP resynthesis.

Fuels for aerobic ATP resynthesis

The two fuels normally utilized by the aerobic mechanism of ATP resynthesis are glycogen and fatty acids. Proteins are only used as fuels when glycogen is lacking, as in starvation or occasionally in endurance events.

Glycogen is a roughly spherical molecule composed of millions of glucose molecules bonded in a tree-like structure (Fig. 1.13). It is present primarily in the muscle and liver cells. The dimension of the glycogen granules increases with nourishment and decreases with starvation. The glucose units are added to or removed from the millions of extremities exposed on the molecule's surface. When necessary, the enzymes for glycogen breakdown can rapidly remove millions of glucose units, which are readily utilized for ATP resynthesis.

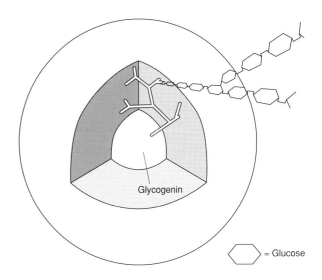

Fig. 1.13 Scheme of the Glycogen molecule.

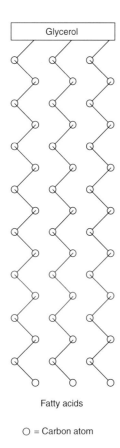

Fig. 1.14 Scheme of a Triglycericle.

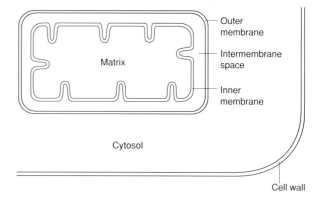

Fig. 1.15 Scheme of a Mitochondrion.

Fatty acids constitute the other combustible that fuels the aerobic mechanism; they are stored as triglycerides mainly in the fat cells, but also in muscle cells (Fig. 1.14). They must be released from glycerol in order to be transported from adipose tissue to the muscles and then inside the mitochondria, where they are broken down.

Site of aerobic ATP resynthesis

Aerobic resynthesis of ATP occurs inside the cells, in organelles called mitochondria. Mitochondria are present in nearly all the cells of the organism in a quantity proportional to their aerobic metabolism. In the heart, for example, which must continuously utilize the aerobic mechanism to resynthesize ATP for its repeated contractions, mitochondria represent one-third of the weight of the organ. Mitochondria

(Fig. 1.15) have a rod-like shape and are covered externally by a continuous membrane. A second membrane, inside the first, has numerous folds called cristae. Fuel breakdown takes place in the core (matrix) of the mitochondria, and ATP resynthesis on the inner membrane.

Process of aerobic fuel breakdown (Fig. 1.16)

Glucose units, trimmed from glycogen granules, undergo a partial breakdown outside the mitochondria. In this multistep process, known as glycolysis, glucose (a six-carbon molecule) is divided into two units of pyruvate (a three-carbon molecule) and two ATP molecules are synthesized. Successively, the pyruvate produced during glycolysis enters the mitochondria. Here, pyruvate becomes acetate, a two-carbon molecule. The breakdown of fatty acids occurs entirely within the mitochondria, where their long structure is progressively shortened by the sequential removal of acetate molecules. Acetate, derived from the breakdown of both glucose and fatty acids, enters into the Krebs cycle, which is a chain of biochemical reactions that can be described as a breakdown machine, where the two-carbon molecules are broken down into carbon dioxide and hydrogen atoms. Some hydrogen atoms are also generated in reactions preceding the cycle and during glycolysis. The hydrogen atoms are further separated into their components: protons and electrons. The electrons constitute the true fuel for ATP resynthesis; they flow through the mitochondrial inner membrane and release energy which is used to push protons outside the mitochondrial

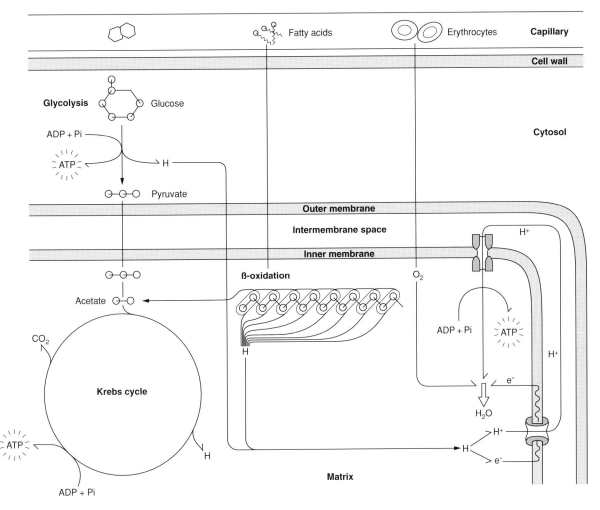

Fig. 1.16 The process of aerobic fuel breakdown.

matrix. Consequently, the proton concentration in the intermembrane space becomes higher than in the matrix. These protons, forced by their higher concentration, then re-enter the matrix with the help of a specific enzyme called ATP-synthase. This proton re-entry flux is utilized to synthesize ATP. Aerobic breakdown of 1 mol of glucose and 1 mol of palmitate, the most common fatty acid in the cells, produces 39 and 129 mol of ATP, respectively. Fatty acids ($C_{16}H_{32}O_2$) generate more ATP than glucose ($C_6H_{12}O_6$) because they contain more hydrogen atoms and thus more electrons, that is, more fuel for ATP resynthesis.

Rate of aerobic ATP resynthesis (aerobic power)

Under resting conditions, the rates of both ATP degradation and resynthesis are low. With an increase in exercise intensity, both rates increase; thus, the rate of fuel breakdown also rises. The mixture of fatty acids and glucose changes with exercise intensity: under resting conditions and low-intensity exercise, fatty acids are the primary fuel, while glucose breakdown augments progressively as exercise intensity increases. In laboratory tests that bring about the full activation of the aerobic mechanism, the maximal rate of aerobic ATP resynthesis can be reached and measured indirectly, through determination of O_2

consumption. The two variables are correlated; thus, the maximal rate of aerobic ATP resynthesis can be calculated indirectly from $V_{O_{2max}}$.

For every litre of O_2 consumed (which burns 1.35 g of glucose), 161.16 g of ATP is resynthesized, more than three times the total amount available within the muscle. In elite athletes, $V_{O_{2max}}$ ranges from 5 to 7 l $O_2 \cdot min^{-1}$, yielding from 806 to 1128 g of ATP per min.

Aerobic power, that is, the maximal rate of ATP resynthesis that a subject can attain while doing a given exercise, depends on the mitochondrial O_2 availability and, even more so, on the amount of O_2 transported to the active muscles by the cardio-circulatory system.

Aerobic endurance and glycogen stores (Fig. 1.17)

Both athletes who race long distances and those who specialize in races lasting only a few minutes (e.g. 1500 m) rely on a powerful aerobic mechanism.

Nevertheless, the short-distance athletes are unable to perform well in long races (e.g. marathons) because they lack aerobic endurance, that is, the ability to sustain high-intensity exercise for a long time.

Aerobic endurance depends on the individual's glycogen stores. During exercise, when glycogen stores become depleted, performance is significantly impaired because the aerobic mechanism then relies on the breakdown of fatty acids. This results in a reduced rate of ATP resynthesis. For example, an athlete who consumes 6 l $O_2 \cdot min^{-1}$ will synthesize 967 g ATP $\cdot min^{-1}$ when burning glucose and only 831.6 g $\cdot min^{-1}$ when burning fatty acids, with about a 14% reduction in aerobic power.

In addition, the exhaustion of glycogen stores reduces the efficiency of the Krebs cycle. Under normal conditions, the cycle continuously loses some of its components. These losses may be counteracted by a restocking reaction based on pyruvate availability. Pyruvate is formed from the breakdown of glucose,

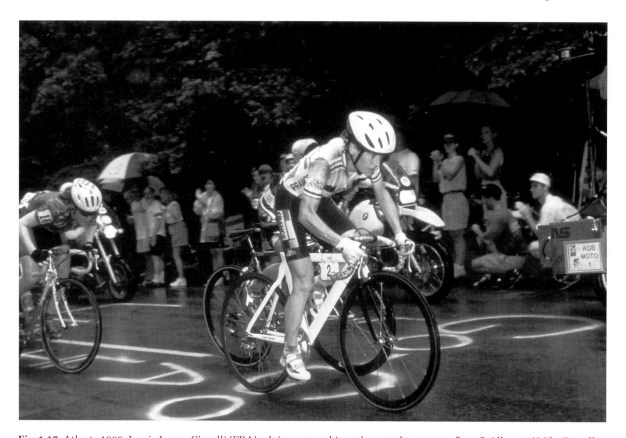

Fig. 1.17 Atlanta 1996. Jeanie Longo-Ciprelli (FRA) relying on aerobic endurance for success, first. © Allsport / Mike Powell.

which in turn derives from glycogen. Therefore, under conditions of glycogen depletion, less pyruvate is available and the Krebs cycle is impoverished. Consequently, less acetate enters the cycle and the rate of ATP resynthesis is further reduced (see Fig. 1.16). An endurance athlete, such as a road-racing cyclist, has about 450 g of glycogen at the race's start: 350 g in the muscles and 100 g in the liver. This quantity is insufficient to cover the several hours of high work intensity required to finish the race. To complete a physical effort of this magnitude, the endurance athlete trains so that muscles make greater use of fatty acids, thereby sparing glycogen. In contrast, athletes who train for shorter events and untrained individuals at the same relative exercise intensity use glycogen almost exclusively and deplete their stores more quickly; thus, they have less aerobic endurance.

In addition to having the physical capacity to spare glycogen, endurance athletes employ racing strategies to avoid using the anaerobic mechanism, which consumes glycogen 13 times faster. Moreover, they reintegrate glycogen reserves through adequate food intake before, during and after the race.

Anaerobic lactacid mechanism of ATP resynthesis

This process of ATP resynthesis involves the same extramitochondrial reactions as aerobic breakdown of glucose, which forms pyruvate (Fig. 1.16). When anaerobic glycolysis is activated, the rate of pyruvate production exceeds the mitochondrial capacity to absorb it. An example is the initial phase of physical activity, when the extramitochondrial phases of glucose breakdown are activated more rapidly than the mitochondrial phases. Another example is of maximal exercise intensity, when glucose breakdown exceeds the mitochondrial capacity to absorb pyruvate. Under these conditions, part of the pyruvate generated by glycolysis does not enter the mitochondria for additional demolition and 'stagnates' in the cell cytoplasm. In addition, part of the hydrogen liberated in one of the extramitochondrial reactions cannot be transferred to the mitochondria for ATP production and is absorbed by pyruvate, which is thus transformed into lactate. The accumulation of lactate signals that some glucose molecules have been broken down anaerobically (anaerobic lactacid glycolysis).

Anaerobic breakdown of a molecule of glucose allows for the resynthesis of 3 mol of ATP when glucose is derived from glycogen, and 2 mol of ATP when starting directly from glucose (glucose found in the blood; using this glucose consumes 1 mol of ATP).

Rate of anaerobic lactacid ATP resynthesis (anaerobic lactacid power)

Although anaerobic glycolysis produces only 3 mol of ATP as opposed to the 39 mol generated when glucose is broken down aerobically, the maximal rate of ATP resynthesis of the anaerobic lactacid mechanism is greater than that of the aerobic mechanism. In fact, full activation of anaerobic glycolysis (e.g. in a prolonged sprint) allows the athlete to reach significantly higher speeds than those obtained in efforts based on the full activation of the aerobic mechanism (e.g. in a time trial).

The anaerobic threshold

At a certain exercise intensity, the rate of ATP breakdown exceeds the rate of aerobic ATP resynthesis. The balance between ATP breakdown and resynthesis is nevertheless maintained, thanks to the activation of anaerobic lactacid ATP resynthesis. The exercise intensity (which varies between individuals) at which anaerobic resynthesis is activated is called the anaerobic threshold. At exercise intensities above the anaerobic threshold, lactate accumulates.

Determination of the anaerobic threshold has practical implications because there is a closer correlation between the anaerobic threshold and aerobic performance than there is with $V_{O_{2max}}$. In addition, training produces more modifications to the aerobic threshold than it does to $V_{O_{2max}}$. Therefore, determination of the anaerobic threshold is more often used in designing training programmes and in evaluating their effects.

Anaerobic lactacid endurance

Anaerobic breakdown of glucose, being much faster but less efficient than its aerobic counterpart, consumes glucose at a high rate. Its maximal employment, for even a few minutes, drastically reduces muscle glycogen reserves, thereby limiting not only aerobic endurance (see above) but also anaerobic endurance, that is, the capacity to perform prolonged maximal work based on the use of anaerobic glycolysis. A second limiting factor in the use of anaerobic glycolysis is lactate accumulation. The subsequent acidification reduces the efficiency of the various muscular functions, including glycolysis and anaerobic ATP resynthesis. The fact that muscular acidification is better withstood by sprinters than by endurance athletes, that is, by subjects having a high percentage of fast-twitch fibres, suggests the importance of genetics in determining anaerobic endurance. Other factors that come into play are the rapidity of lactate diffusion in the extracellular spaces and in the blood, its subsequent removal from the blood by the liver and heart and also of its reuse by the muscles

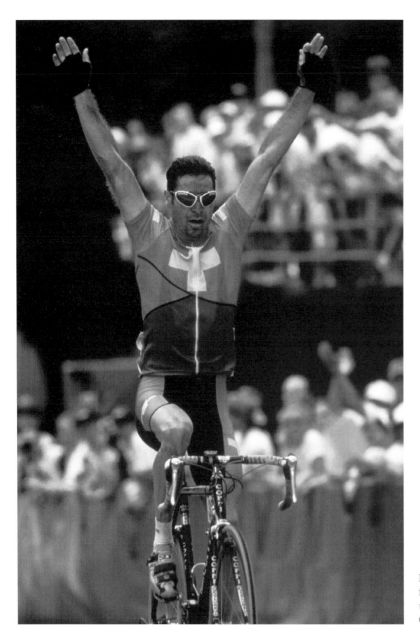

Fig. 1.18 Atlanta 1996: road race. The finish and victory of Richard Pascal, using an efficient metabolic system. © Allsport / Pascal Rondeau.

(immediately or in the recovery phase of an anaerobic workout). Anaerobic lactacid endurance varies between individuals. Some cyclists are able to employ the anaerobic lactacid mechanism longer and without an appreciable drop in power. For the same glycogen availability, these athletes are more able than others to resist lactate acidification, probably due to a better buffering system or faster lactate removal (Fig. 1.18, p. 16).

Physiology and biochemistry of various types of cyclists

Road cycling requires the combined use of all three mechanisms of ATP resynthesis. However, varieties in racing terrain and distance favour athletes having different mixtures of these mechanisms.

Sprinters

These athletes are able to reach very high pedalling cadences (180 rpm or more) and speeds (70 km/hr or more) for a few seconds in the final sprint. They possess great muscle mass, especially the quadriceps, and high anaerobic alactacid power. In 10-sec all-out tests, their peak power can exceed 1500 W, and their average power 1300 W. Not having a very highly developed aerobic mechanism, they can excel in races that are not very demanding and in which the finish is on the flats.

Finisseurs

These athletes are able to maintain speeds considerably above their AT for a relatively long time (a few minutes). They possess a greater than average power and, above all, endurance of the anaerobic lactacid mechanism. Their average power output in 30-s all-out tests exceeds 1000 W. They excel for example in races that finish with a 1–2 km climb.

Time trialists

These athletes are able to maintain a fast pace for a long period (about one hour). They usually have a large physical stature, with very high Vo_{2max} and a power output at AT sometimes exceeding 500 W. They possess a greater than average aerobic power and excel in time trial events. Some elite time trialists have a smaller physical stature and less aerobic power but superior aerodynamic characteristics.

Climbers

These athletes are usually of small physical stature and light weight and excel in long climbs, which involve the aerobic mechanism. Although they do not possess high aerobic power in absolute terms (less than 400 W at AT), their weight-to-aerobic power ratio is much greater than average (higher than 6 W/kg at AT). While climbing they are able to push big gears and to change pace easily.

Chapter 2

Biomechanics of road cycling

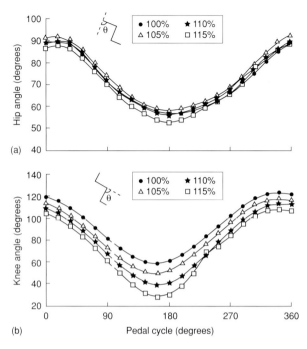

(a)

(b)

Fig. 2.1 Angular displacement of (a) the hip and (b) the knee for one pedalling cycle at four different seat heights at 100, 105, 110 and 115% of leg length. Reprinted with permission from Gregor and Fowler (1996).

Cycling kinematics

The reference frame used in Chapter 1 to discuss muscle activity patterns with respect to crank rotation in the pedalling cycle will be used again in this chapter to describe lower-extremity kinematics and kinetics. As before, the power or propulsive phase takes place between 0° (top dead centre) and 180° (bottom dead centre) in the pedalling cycle. From 180° of crank rotation back to 360° constitutes the recovery phase; when the right lower extremity is in the propulsive phase, the left lower extremity is in recovery.

Most reports on cycling kinematics have been limited to sagittal plane motion: hip and knee flexion and extension and ankle dorsiflexion and plantar flexion. Displacements, velocities and accelerations of the thigh, shank and foot seem to be most affected by cadence and bicycle geometry – seat height, crank length and foot position on the pedal. The complex interactions between bicycle geometry and rider kinematics and attempts to optimize the bicycle–rider system have been the subject of many studies which systematically varied rider kinematics by changing either bicycle configuration or pedalling cadence or both. Peak flexion and extension of the lower-extremity joints will vary depending on the seat height and fore–aft adjustments. However, once the constrained cyclic movement of the lower extremity is established for comfort by each rider at a selected seat position and crank length, lower-extremity kinematic patterns remain quite consistent.

When a seat height is chosen for comfort by the individual cyclist, the range of motion reported for the thigh is approximately 45° from maximum flexion to maximum extension. The range of motion of the knee is slightly larger and averages about 75° from

maximum flexion to maximum extension, while the ankle has a more limited range of motion with a total excursion of approximately 20° between maximum dorsiflexion and maximum plantar flexion. Range-of-motion data for the hip and knee are presented in Fig. 2.1. These data show the effect of seat height on hip and knee range of motion. The seat height varied from 100 to 115% of the pubic symphysis height (height measured from the pubic symphysis, or crotch, to the floor). Essentially, there was little difference in the hip range of motion across the four seat heights, while knee range of motion did change, but the general pattern remained the same. The hip extension range varys from 90° down to 50°, while the knee extension range starts at 120° and drops down to between 30° and 60°. The range of seat heights presented in this figure is considered somewhat extreme, since the comfortable range chosen by most competitive riders usually varies from 106 to 109% of the public symphysis height. Similar investigations have been conducted using seat height conditions of between 94 and 106% of pubic symphysis height.

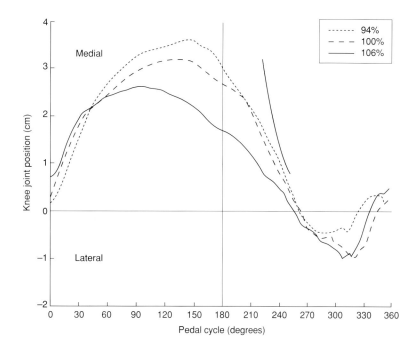

Fig. 2.2 Knee position during the pedalling cycle with respect to the pedal centre of pressure at three different seat heights: 94, 100 and 106% of leg length. Each curve is an average of 150 pedal revolutions at 200 W and 80 rpm. Reproduced with permission from McCoy (1989).

Using these seat-height conditions, almost identical results at the knee and the hip were reported. In all of the data, however, the knee seem to be the joint which is most affected by changes in seat height.

While movements in the sagittal plane – hip, knee and ankle flexion and extension – dominate during the cycling task, considerable movement has been reported outside the sagittal plane to involve both the transverse and frontal planes. For example, internal and external rotation of the tibia (about its long axis), knee translation in the frontal plane (movement of the knee toward and away from the bicycle) and considerable movement of the lower extremity outside the sagittal plane have all been presented in a variety of articles, both scientific and popular. Data presented in Fig. 2.2 indicate considerable medial and lateral movement of the knee joint. Beginning at 0° or dead centre, the knee moves from a neutral position towards the bicycle and reaches its maximum medial position after 90° of crank rotation. The knee then moves laterally to reach a maximum lateral position at approximately 300° of crank rotation. It is also apparent from Fig. 2.2 that seat height has a considerable effect on the medial and lateral movement of the knee. The lower the seat height, the greater the medial movement and the later in the pedalling cycle peak that the

medial position is reached. It seems that the highest saddle position had the least amount of medial translation of the knee towards the bicycle in the power phase. This pattern of knee movement has been reported by several investigators.

At this point it is fitting to ask: How much movement should be allowed before muscle and connective tissue structures are so stressed or strained that injury may occur? Several investigators have reported that subjects without knee problems display less medial lateral movement of the knee. In support of these facts, investigators have used qualitative video analysis and reported less knee movement in the frontal plane in elite cyclists using in-shoe orthotics. Trial-and-error adjustment in pedal cant and video feedback reduction in frontal plane movement seem to reduce knee pain in elite cyclists. How much to limit natural movement of the lower-extremity structures remains open to debate. Consequently, caution should be exercised when selecting information from investigations and applying it to personal performance.

As discussed in Chapter 1, muscle length has an effect on the ability to produce force. As a consequence of movement in the lower extremity during cycling, leg muscles continuously change length. In addition, the velocity at which these muscles move

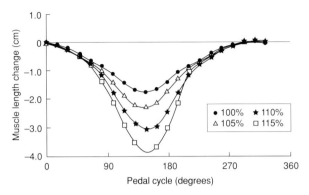

Fig. 2.3 Patterns of muscle length change during the pedalling cycle for the vasti group (vastus lateralis and medialis). Data are for four different seat heights: 100, 105, 110 and 115% of leg length. The zero line represents the muscle length with the hip and knee at 90° and negative slopes indicate muscle shortening. Reprinted with permission from Gregor and Fowler (1996).

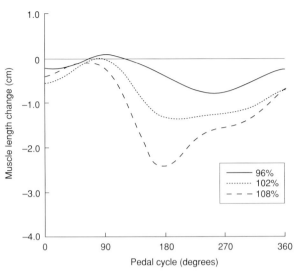

Fig. 2.4 Pattern of muscle length for the soleus muscle during the pedalling cycle at three different seat heights: 96, 102 and 108% of leg length. The zero line represents the muscle length in the normal standing position and negative slopes indicate muscle shortening. Reprinted with permission from Gregor and Fowler (1996).

also varies during the pedalling cycle. It is important to understand the length change patterns of the muscles in the lower extremity during cycling in order to understand, firstly, how muscle contributes to energizing the bicycle, and secondly, how much the muscle can stretch and the risk of injury.

Using hip, knee and ankle joint range-of-motion data and lower-extremity anatomy, estimates of muscle length changes for many of the major lower-extremity muscle tendon units have been made. Fig. 2.3 presents data on changes in the length of the vasti group as a function of change in seat height from 100 to 115% of the pubic symphysis height.

These single-joint knee extensors have similar patterns of length change across the four seat height conditions, but show peak stretch on the muscle at approximately bottom dead centre in the pedalling cycle at all four seat-height conditions. The greatest range of length change was experienced at the 115% seat height, where the muscles stretched approximately 4 cm. While we do not know the effect of this calculated length change on sarcomere spacing, we do know that seat height has a marked effect on the stretch and shortening of this muscle group.

Similar to the single-joint knee extensor, the single-joint ankle extensor – the soleus muscle – was markedly affected by seat-height changes. In Fig. 2.4, data are presented at three seat-height conditions,

varying from 96 to 108% of the pubic symphysis height. Clearly, the greatest amount of lengthening occurred at 108% seat height. At all seat-height conditions, the muscle was observed to stretch slightly until about 90° of crank rotation and to then markedly shorten, reaching a peak at both 102 and 108% seat-height conditions at approximately bottom dead centre. The least amount of shortening which would result from plantar flexion of the ankle was observed at 96% seat height.

Unlike the single-joint muscles, muscles crossing adjacent joints are affected by the movement and range of motion of the adjacent joints. For example, the hamstring muscles are affected by movement at the hip and at the knee, since they extend the hip and flex the knee. Consequently, the range of motion experienced by the hip and knee in combination will have an effect on the length change of the hamstring group. Data for hamstring length changes at four different seat-height positions, to include 100–115% of pubic symphysis height, are presented in Fig. 2.5. It can be observed that the hamstrings stretch slightly early in the pedalling cycle, but that most of the pedalling cycle is devoted to muscle shortening. Peak

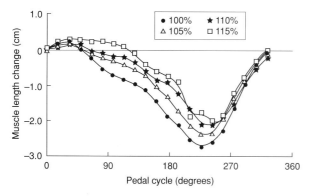

Fig. 2.5 Pattern of muscle length change during the pedalling cycle for the hamstring group (all biarticular muscles) at four different seat heights: 100, 105, 110 and 115% of leg length. The zero line represents the muscle length with the hip and knee at 90° and negative slopes indicate muscle shortening. Reprinted with permission from Gregor and Fowler (1996).

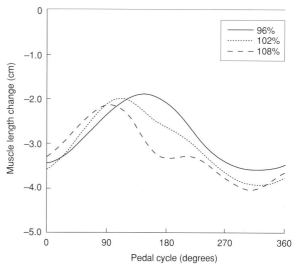

Fig. 2.6 Pattern of muscle length change during the pedalling cycle for the biarticular gastrocnemius muscle (both medial and lateral heads) at three different seat heights: 96, 102 and 108% leg length. The zero line represents the muscle length in the normal standing position and negative slopes indicate muscle shortening. Reprinted with permission from Gregor and Fowler (1996).

shortening distances are observed at approximately 270° of crank rotation. Essentially, then, in the fourth quadrant, or from 270° to 360°, the muscles in the hamstring group begin to stretch again. Seat height does have an effect on the absolute changes in muscle length in the hamstring group, and it should be remembered that this continuous stretch/shortening cycle of the muscle will have an effect on its force output.

Similar to the biarticular hamstring group, length changes in the two-joint gastrocnemius are also affected by seat-height position. Patterns of stretch and subsequent shortening are noticed at each seat height presented in Fig. 2.6. While seat height affected the absolute length changes in the hamstring group, more than the gastrocnemius, the 108% seat-height condition was noticeably different from the other two seat-height conditions for the gastrocnemius. In general, the gastrocnemius stretches for the first 90° of the pedalling cycle, reaching a peak somewhere in the middle of the second quadrant. The time of peak stretch on the gastrocnemius was related to seat height, as was the rate of shortening. The slope of the 108% seat-height condition was much steeper than the slope at the 102 and 96% seat-height condition. As discussed previously, muscle lengthening and shortening velocities will also affect the muscle's ability to produce a force.

Evaluating the data presented in Figs 2.3–2.6, these patterns of muscle-length changes were fairly consistent and have been supported by many reports in the literature. One final noticeable difference in the length-change patterns between the biarticular and single-joint muscles shows that single-joint muscles appear to be affected more by seat-height conditions and changed their length to a greater degree than the biarticular muscles. For example, the single-joint knee extensors, i.e. the vasti group, have a length change of approximately 4 cm at the highest seat height, while the hamstring group has a length change of only 2.5–3 cm. The soleus muscle, at the highest seat-height condition, has a length change of approximately 2.5 cm, while the gastrocnemius muscle has a length change of only 2 cm. The fact that biarticular muscles are not stretched as much as uniarticular muscles also leads us to believe that the velocities of shortening in uniarticular muscles will be higher than those in biarticular muscles. These data have direct implications on flexibility, on exercises for the lower extremity, and on any training related to enhancing the participation of lower-extremity musculature, whether specifically a single-joint muscle or a biarticular muscle.

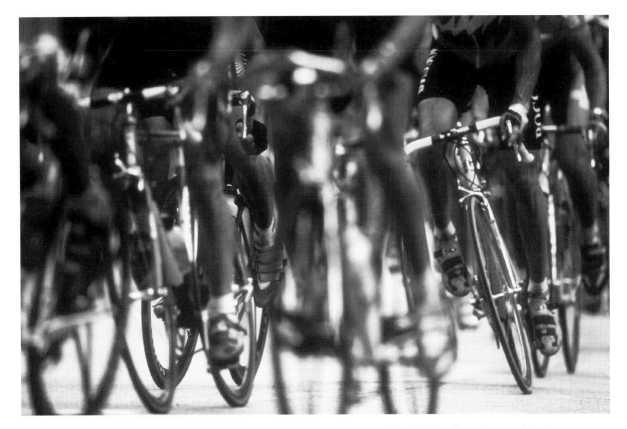

Fig. 2.7 Atlanta 1996, depicting the legs, the most significant energy source to drive the bicycle. © Allsport / Stu Forster.

Cycling kinetics (Fig. 2.7)

Pedal reaction forces

Mechanical analysis of lower-extremity function during cycling requires knowledge of the interactive forces between the rider and the bicycle. When the foot applies a force to the pedal, it will be met with a reaction force that is equal in magnitude and opposite in direction. These forces, called pedal reaction forces, act on the lower limb during cycling and have been quantified by use of specially instrumented pedals (see Fig. 2.14). Force components perpendicular to the pedal surface (Fz), as well as shear forces paralleled to the pedal surface, both medial lateral (Fx) and anterior/posterior (Fy) (Fig. 2.8a), have been measured, and from these components a centre of pressure (Fig. 2.8c, Ay and Ax) or point of force application can be calculated. Finally, a rotational

moment about an axis perpendicular to the surface of the pedal (Fig. 2.8b, Mz, Fig. 2.14) and positioned at the centre of pressure may also be quantified. This rotational moment will be discussed later in this chapter.

The perpendicular component of the pedal reaction force were first reported in 1896 by A. Sharp in a book entitled *Bicycles and Tricycles*. However, it was not until 70 years later that this subject was reported again. Subsequently, results of a two-dimensional force pedal analysis were presented in numerous studies and all follow the same pattern presented in Fig. 2.8(a). As observed in Fig. 2.8(a), peak force perpendicular to the pedal surface (Fz) is approximately 350 N or 60% of the subject's body weight. This percentage is about the same for all seated cycling under steady-state conditions. These reaction forces will, of course, increase as resistance increases but rarely exceed body weight unless the subject stands up during sprinting or climbing. In addition, while riders often feel that they pull up on the pedals during recovery, this is rare and most riders usually do not do so. Pulling up on the pedal is not essential to an efficient cycling technique and competitive riders reserve this action for climbing or sprinting. Finally, symmetry in pedalling technique is also rare. This is true for both highly competitive and recreational cyclists. Depending on power requirements, individual conditioning and bike set-up, bilateral asymmetry can be pronounced.

While the magnitude of the pedal reaction force is important, the orientation of the resultant vector (Fr) with respect to the lower extremity is also important and will markedly influence how the leg musculature responds to varying demands. An exemplar pattern of the resultant pedal reaction force measured at six intervals during the pedalling cycle is presented in Fig. 2.9, together with the relationship between the resultant vector and the right lower extremity. In this example, if the force vector is in front of the hip centre of rotation, then the hip extensor muscles will be activated to counterbalance the force coming from the pedal. If the same force vector is behind the centre of rotation for the knee, then the knee extensor muscles will be activated to counterbalance this force coming from the pedal. And finally, if the force vector is in front of the ankle joint, the plantar flexors will be activated by the nervous system to counterbalance the force vector coming from the pedal.

While the position of this force vector in the sagittal plane will dictate involvement of hip, knee and ankle flexors and extensors, movement of this force vector in the frontal plane, or medial lateral plane, will affect muscle activity related to adduction and abduction. As indicated in Fig. 2.10, the resultant vector is medial to the knee joint for almost all of the power phase. This is true at medium and high seat height, but not true when lower seat heights are used (94% of pubic symphysis height). While the data are inconsistent across seat heights, it is apparent from the information presented in Fig. 2.10 that during the recovery phase of the pedalling cycle (180–360°), the resultant force vector is lateral to the knee. These data have been

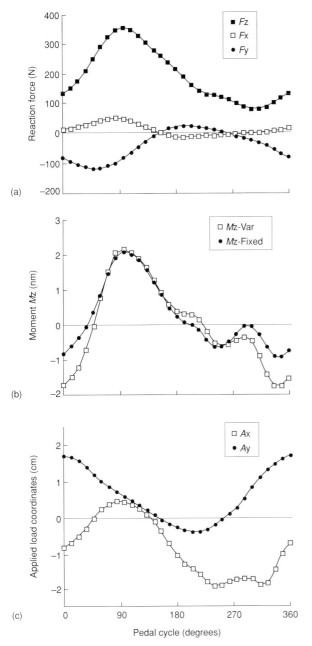

(a)

(b)

(c)

Fig. 2.8 Average patterns for five pedal revolutions: (a) pedal reaction force, (b) applied moment and (c) centre of pressure during one pedalling cycle. (a) Fz, force component at 90° to the pedal surface; Fy, shear component along the pedal surface; Fx, shear component in the medial lateral direction. (b) Mz, applied moment about an axis perpendicular to the pedal surface and located at the centre of pressure (Mz-VAR) or through the centre of the pedal (mz-fixed). (c) Coordinates of the applied load in the x and y direction. Reproduced with permission from Broker and Gregor (1990).

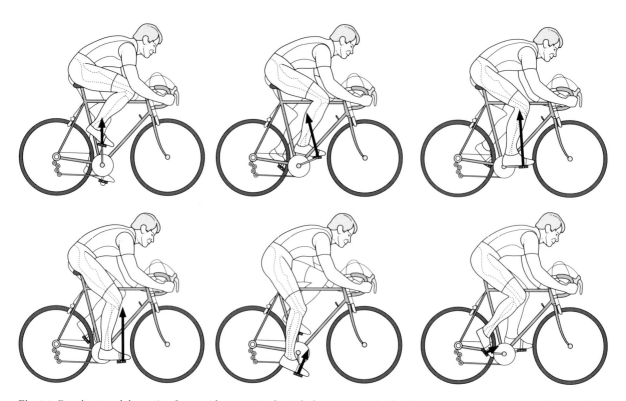

Fig. 2.9 Resultant pedal reaction force with respect to the right lower extremity for six separate locations during the pedalling cycle. The length of the arrow indicates increases and decreases in force magnitude.

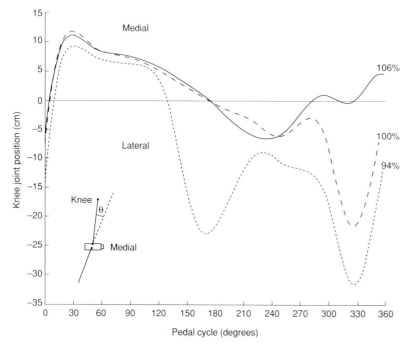

Fig. 2.10 Position of the pedal reaction force with respect to the knee during the pedalling cycle in the frontal plane. Each curve is an average of 150 pedal revolutions at 200 W and 80 rpm. Separate patterns are an average at three seat conditions: 94, 100 and 106% of leg length. Reproduced with permission from McCoy (1989).

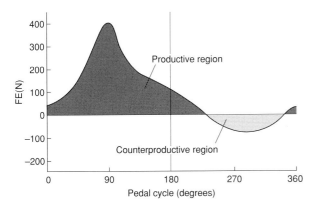

Fig. 2.11 Effective force profile during one pedal revolution. productive region is positive work performed to drive the crank in a clockwise direction while the counterproductive region (during recovery) represents work done against the crank to rotate it in an anticlockwise direction. Reprinted with permission from Gregor and Fowler (1996).

reported by several authors, and it can be concluded that seat-height variations affect the range of motion of the lower extremity in both the sagittal and frontal planes. In turn this will affect the position of the force vector coming from the pedal with respect to hip, knee and ankle joint position.

One final observation with respect to the forces acting on the pedal and subsequently acting on the crank to power the bicycle relates to how effective the forces are when applied to the pedal and crank in energizing the bicycle. An effective force is a force component perpendicular to the crank, and an ineffective force is a component parallel to the crank which has no effect on crank rotation, and subsequently no effect on energizing the bicycle. The ratio between the effective and ineffective force components has been described as the index of effectiveness.

Information presented in Fig. 2.11 indicates the maximum effective force component applied to the crank during the power phase. In addition, during recovery, ineffective forces may act on the crank and reduce the rider's efficiency. Elite riders, in general, have a high index of effectiveness which appears to be unaffected by their position on the bicycle. In other words, if elite cyclists or triathletes assume an aerodynamic versus an advanced aerodynamic position, their index of effectiveness generally remains un-

changed. Finally, the type of shoe–pedal interface – whether toe strap and cleat, clipless fixed or clipless float – had little effect on the power transmitted to the bike as measured by the effective crank force patterns. This is a significant result since there has been speculation that certain types of pedals will reduce power transmitted to the bicycle. There are no data to support this speculation.

Pedal pressure distribution

Thus far, we have discussed the resultant pedal reaction force and its importance when studying lower-extremity muscle involvement and energizing the bicycle. While it is useful to study a single point of force application on the pedal, in reality pressures are distributed over the sole of the shoe as it interacts with the pedal during the pedalling cycle. A typical pattern of pressure distribution is presented in Fig. 2.12. The magnitude of the pressure is directly affected by the amount of force applied to the pedal. The area of highest pressure concentration is influenced by how the foot interacts with the shoe against the pedal as well as by the type of pedal and the type of shoe, e.g. soft-soled or hard-soled shoes. There are many reports in the scientific literature which support the pattern of pressure presented in Fig. 2.12. Almost all the pressure is concentrated beneath the large toe and little pressure is exerted at the arch or heel or on the lateral side of the foot. It should be remembered, however, that this distribution will change as a function of shoe and pedal type.

Joint reaction forces

We have evaluated the function of the lower extremity, so far, with respect to muscle activity patterns, subsequent forces produced by those muscles and the reaction forces produced at the shoe–pedal interface. Much of the scientific literature evaluates lower-extremity function during different forms of cycling by modelling the leg as a system of linked rigid bodies. The thigh, leg and foot are considered to be three segments interacting to achieve a common objective – to impart power to the crank. If muscles produce internal forces, and the pedal–foot interface provides an environmental reaction force on the plantar surface of the foot, then forces are also

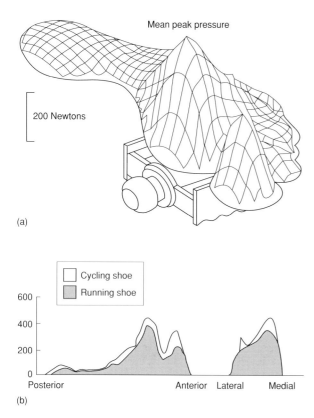

Mean peak pressure

200 Newtons

(a)

☐ Cycling shoe
▨ Running shoe

600

400

200

0

Posterior   Anterior   Lateral   Medial

(b)

Fig. 2.12 (a) Pattern of pressure distribution on the sole of the shoe, including data from a subject using a cycling shoe and a running shoe (b). Reproduced with permission from Sanderson (1990).

experienced within the joints of the leg. These reaction forces, produced in the joints of the lower extremity – the hip, knee and ankle – are generally referred to as joint reaction forces. Since the bicycle is used both for exercise and competition, as well as rehabilitation, the most commonly reported data on joint reaction forces relate to the knee. While details can be found in the scientific literature, the following summary can be made:

1 During the power phase, there is a compressive joint reaction force produced by the distal end of the femur on the tibial plateau.

2 There is an anteriorly directed joint reaction force throughout the power phase regardless of seat-height position.

3 There is a laterally directed joint reaction force at the knee throughout the power phase regardless of seat-height position.

Peak joint reaction forces, whether anteriorly directed, laterally directed or compressive, have their highest value at approximately 90° of the pedalling cycle.

Muscle moment patterns

This section is devoted to the calculation of muscle moments during the cycling task. The muscle moment represents a summation or integration of all active and passive components that will produce a force about a joint in an attempt to rotate that joint into, for example, flexion or extension. Contributors to these muscle moments include individual muscle forces, ligament forces and passive tendon forces. Each of the forces produced by these various tissues in the lower extremity acts at some distance from an axis of rotation and attempts to rotate the joint in the direction in which the force is applied. Since the calculation of a muscle moment at the joint represents a summation of all the individual forces, it is important to know how individual muscles act at certain phases of the pedalling cycle, and which muscles, by virtue of their electrical activity, dominate in their control of limb position. We must also remember, as discussed previously, that some muscles cross a single joint and affect only that joint, while other muscles cross two joints and affect two adjacent joints simultaneously. In other words, a biarticular muscle will contribute to the muscle moment calculated at the two adjacent joints simultaneously. The rectus femoris, if activated, will contribute to the muscle moment calculated at the hip as well as the muscle moment calculated at the knee.

The patterns of joint moments presented for the ankle, knee and hip in Fig. 2.13 have been supported by a wide variety of reports in the literature. These muscle moment patterns are easily repeated despite variations in loading conditions, subject population and bike set-up. Magnitudes increase in response to increased environmental demands, and some of the timing features may be affected by cadence and whether the rider is accelerating into a sprint or just riding comfortably at a constant cadence. However, in almost all cases, the general patterns presented in Fig. 2.13 remain the same.

The muscle moment calculated at the ankle is always a plantar flexor moment through the power phase and into most of the recovery phase. This moment represents dominance of the ankle plantar flexors attempting to plantarflex the ankle against the reaction force coming from the pedal on the plantar surface of the foot. In other words, the reaction force from the pedal attempts to dorsiflex the foot, while the muscles in the posterior compartment of the leg, i.e. the plantar flexors, counteract this environmental force and attempt to plantarflex the foot. Since this muscle moment represents the activity of all active and passive structures surrounding the ankle, a plantar flexor muscle moment is calculated.

The muscle moment calculated at the hip is almost always extensor through most of the power phase into the recovery phase. In some cases there is a small portion of the recovery phase dedicated to a hip flexor moment. It can be seen from Fig. 2.13 that the variability in magnitude of the hip extensor moment in the power phase is considerable. These data indicate that hip extensors are active in counteracting the pedal reaction force. Despite the fact that the hip goes into extension during the power phase and flexes during recovery for most of the pedalling cycle, the muscle moment calculated at the hip is extensor.

The knee is very different from the ankle and the hip in its muscle moment profile during the pedalling cycle. During the power phase the knee extends to bottom dead centre and then flexes from 180° to 360° of the pedalling cycle. The pattern presented in Fig. 2.13 shows that the knee muscle moment is extensor until just after 90° in the pedalling cycle and then becomes flexor for almost all the rest of the pedalling cycle. This means that the musculature surrounding the knee attempts to extend the knee until approximately 100° in the pedalling cycle and then attempts to flex the knee for the remainder of the power phase and into recovery. The significance of this information is discussed on many occasions in the scientific literature. Also, the relationship between muscle activity patterns and these muscle moment patterns, calculated using engineering mechanics, is quite complex. Consequently, the reader is again referred to the extensive scientific literature describing this relationship.

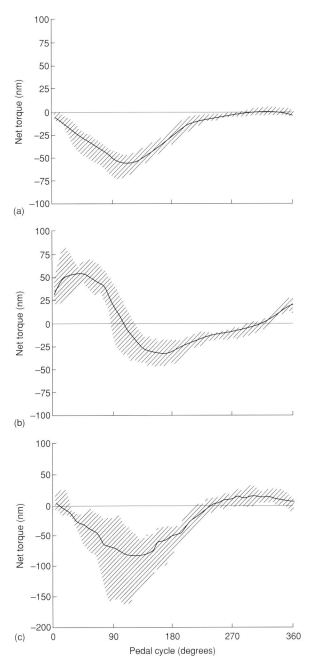

Fig. 2.13 Muscle moment (torque) patterns for (a) the ankle, (b) the knee and (c) the hip during the pedalling cycle. Data represent an average of 25 pedalling cycles at approximately 260 W and 84 rpm. Reproduced with permission from Gregor, Cavanagh and La Fortune (1985).

Shoe–pedal interface

Knowledge of torsion or rotation of segments about a long axis through the centre of the segment is important to understand musculoskeletal function and, in particular, mechanisms of injury. Because of the significance of this rotation, its relationship to injury and its similarities in cycling and running, there are several reports in the literature on this topic. In order to investigate segment rotations during cycling and their potential relationship to injury, one particular measurement must be made at the shoe–pedal interface. This measurement relates to an applied moment at the pedal surface about an axis perpendicular to the pedal surface. A sketch of this type of calculation is presented in Fig. 2.14. It can be seen that if the rider attempts to rotate the foot internally as it pushes on the pedal, a positive torsion moment will result. If he or she attempts to rotate the foot outward against the pedal, there is a negative torsional moment. Specifically, inward rotation means that the heel moves away from the midline and away from the bicycle and in outward rotation the heel moves towards the midline or the frame of the bicycle. This calculation is especially important when discussing the different types

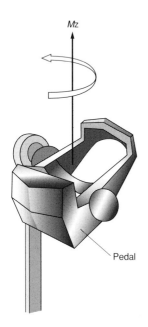

Fig. 2.14 Sketch of the applied moment (*Mz*) about an axis perpendicular to the pedal surface.

of shoe–pedal interface, and whether the leg is allowed to rotate freely in a float clipless design or constrained in a more limited range of motion.

Data presented in Fig. 2.15(a) show the results of this pedal torsion calculation when using a toe strap and cleat, a clipless fixed and a clipless float pedal design. Across a wide range of subjects, it was seen that the fixed clipless design had the highest peak torsional moment. This moment reached its peak at approximately 90° of the pedalling cycle. Fig. 2.15(b) shows the pattern of an individual experiencing lateral anterior knee pain. The peak forces experienced by this individual were higher than the average torsional moment calculated for over 30 subjects. This information is relevant to shoe and pedal design, as well as to injury mechanisms and the prevention of injury to cyclists.

From metabolic to mechanical work

In cycling, the efficiency of the transposition of metabolic activity (adenosine triphosphate resynthesis) into exercise intensity (EI) presents important individual differences.

Figure 2.16 shows the relationship between EI and oxygen consumption (Vo_2), as seen in two professional cyclists examined on a wind-load simulator using their own bicycles. As illustrated, at any given Vo_2, the power output differs for the two subjects. For example, at a Vo_2 of 4 l · min^{-1}, one subject's EI is 300 W while the other's is 360 W – a 20% difference. In terms of cycling performance, evaluation of the metabolic activity (aerobic or anaerobic) is therefore less informative than determination of the corresponding EI. However, metabolic testing is useful to monitor the effects of training. Variations in the transformation of metabolic activity into mechanical work depend on the biomechanical characteristics of the subject. Moreover, variations also exist within the same individual; for example, changes in Vo_2 have been shown with modifications in cycling position and pedalling hip angle.

From mechanical work to speed

In Mexico City in 1972, Eddy Merckx rode a classic track bicycle 49.43 km in 1 h, establishing the world hour record at the time. His bicycle had no aero-

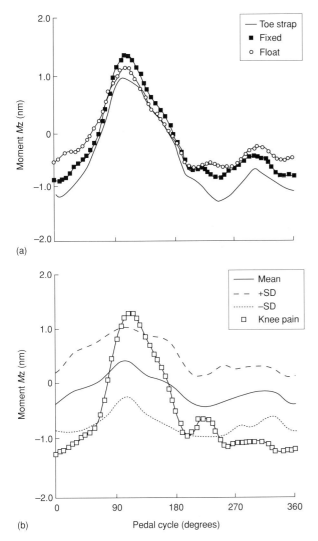

(a)

(b)

Fig. 2.15 The applied moment (*Mz*) pattern during the pedal cycle. (a) Data represent the average of 27 subjects using three separate shoe–pedal interface designs – a standard toe strap and cleat, a clipless fixed design and a clipless float design. A positive moment indicates an inwardly applied moment against the pedal surface (heel out). (b) The pattern of an individual with lateral anterior knee pain (–□–) as well as the mean torsional moment for more than 30 subjects. Reproduced with permission from Wheeler *et al.* (1995).

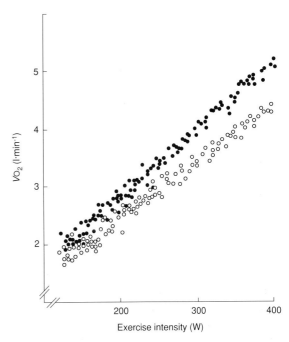

Fig. 2.16 Exercise intensity versus oxygen consumption for two professional cyclists examined using a wind-load simulator and their own bicycles.

dynamic components. Three years later, he rode an ergometer for 1 h in a laboratory in Cologne, Germany, producing an estimated average power output of 455 W (Peronnet *et al.*, 1991), giving coaches and scientists an idea of how great an effort a successful

hour record attempt requires. Fourteen years later, Chris Boardman rode a streamlined bicycle in a stretched-out, superman-like position 55.88 km in 1 h. According to his coach, who regularly monitored Chris with on-board cycling instrumentation, the effort required a continuous power output of nearly 440 W.

The difference between Chris Boardman's and Eddy Merckx's hour record rides – well over two laps on a 250 m track – has little to do with physical capacity to perform work, and everything to do with rider position, bicycle design and optimal integration of rider and bicycle. An equation of motion for each rider would reveal that both balanced external forces with muscular output, and in fact probably performed an equal amount of mechanical work and thus power in their respective efforts. In this section, an equation of motion for a rider and bicycle will be presented and discussed. In particular, the driving forces at the pedal will first be described, explaining how energy flows to the rear wheel in an oscillatory fashion. Next, energy losses between the pedal and rear tyre propulsion point will be examined. Rolling resistance and grade effects will then be discussed. Finally, critical elements of bicycle aerodynamics will be examined, including bicycle design, wheel and component selection, and critical rider positioning effects.

Equation of motion

An equation describing the relationship between rider work and bicycle speed can be developed by considering the five principal resistive elements: drive train friction, inertial forces associated with acceleration of the bicycle, gravitational forces in climbing, tyre rolling resistance and aerodynamic drag. A functional equation of motion for bicycle riding accounting for these five elements takes the form:

$$P_{cyc} = P_{dt} + mVA_{cyc} + WV\sin(\arctan G)$$
$$+ WVCrr_1\cos(\arctan G)$$
$$+ NCrr_2V^2 + 1/2\ C_dA_p\ V(V + V_w)^2$$

where:

P_{cyc} = net instantaneous mechanical power produced by the rider
P_{dt} = power to overcome drive train friction
m = mass of the rider and bicycle
V = bicycle velocity
A_{cyc} = instantaneous acceleration or deceleration of the bicycle–rider system
W = weight of the bicycle and rider
G = the grade
Crr_1 = coefficient of static rolling resistance
N = number of wheels (in case a tricycle is analysed)
Crr_2 = coefficient of dynamic rolling resistance
C_d = coefficient of aerodynamic drag
A_p = frontal surface area of the rider and bicycle
D = air density
V_w = velocity of the head or tail wind (positive for head wind).

In examining the equation above, several important points emerge. Firstly, mass (or weight) of the rider and bicycle figures linearly into the second, third and fourth elements of the equation. That is, a 10% increase in rider plus bicycle weight increases the power required to accelerate the bicycle, power to overcome gravity and power to overcome static rolling resistance by 10%. Power to offset dynamic rolling resistance, the fifth term in the equation above, is

independent of rider and bicycle mass, but increases as the square of bicycle velocity. Finally, power to overcome aerodynamic drag increases as the third power of velocity, so doubling bicycle speed increases power to overcome aerodynamic forces by a factor of eight! As all the elements contribute to the power the rider must produce to maintain forward motion, each element will be discussed in more detail.

Power at the pedals

Figure 2.17 shows, in clock diagram form, the direction and magnitude of the forces a rider applies to the pedals during a typical pedal cycle at 100 rpm and 300 W. These forces were measured on a US national team cyclist by instrumented bicycle pedals. Forces on the pedal through the top of the stroke are small and usually directed slightly forward. Forward-directed forces through the top, accomplished by pushing the toes into the front of the cycling shoes, generate crank torque through this region where power to the cranks is generally low. Peak forces and crank torque occur when the crank is nearly horizontal in the down stroke. Forces through the bottom of the stroke are largely downward, due to gravitational and inertial effects (as the rider's leg motion is changed from downward to upward by the pedal). A slight rearward orientation of the pedal force at the bottom serves to generate crank torque, and thus propel the bicycle. During the upstroke, forces are small and downward, in the opposite direction to the pedal motion. These counter-productive pedal forces

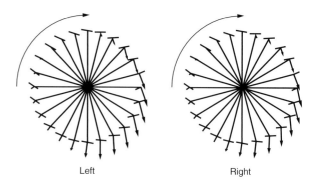

Left   Right

Fig. 2.17 Cycling clock diagrams showing the direction and magnitude of pedal loading for a US national team rider pedalling at 300 W and 100 rpm. Reproduced with permission from Broker and Gregor (1996).

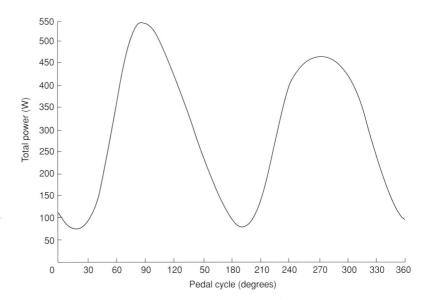

Fig. 2.18 Total power produced by the net effect of forces applied to both pedals. The diagram represents one average revolution of the crank, beginning and ending with the right pedal at the top of the pedal cycle, for a cyclist riding at 300 W and 100 rpm. The first and second peaks occur during the right and left pedal down strokes, respectively. Reproduced with permission from Broker and Gregor (1996).

are nearly always present under steady-state riding conditions, even for elite riders. Muscular actions in this region serve to lift the limb, but not as fast as the pedal is rising.

The net effect of crank torque on both pedals is shown in Fig. 2.18, where total power developed by the rider is plotted versus crank angle. Considerable oscillations occur about the average power of 300 W. Two power peaks are evident, corresponding to the separate peak torque regions for the right and left pedals (when they are near horizontal in the down-stroke). Different magnitudes for the peaks in Fig. 2.18 are due to differences between the peak torques produced at each pedal, and differences in the counter-productive pedal loads during the upstroke. The two minima (valleys) observed in the total power curve represent power-passive periods, occurring when the cranks are near vertical.

Tests with US national team riders in the road, track and mountain bike disciplines reveal that kilometre track specialists and mountain bike racers have the lowest relative oscillations in total power during pedalling. Kilometre specialists must reduce oscillations because average power is well in excess of 1000 W, and thus they must distribute power to the pedal over more of the cycle to avoid extremely high peak powers. Low oscillations in mountain bike racer pedalling mechanics appear to be highly functional as rear wheel traction on loose soil depends in part on continuous and smooth power flow from the pedals.

Drive train power losses

Returning to the equation of motion, energy is delivered to the rear wheel through the chain and transmission elements. Friction in the bottom bracket bearings, chain elements and rear transmission consumes a small portion of this energy. Tests by Danh *et al.* (1991) and Kyle (1988) indicate that cone and cup bearings have one-seventh the friction of cartridge bearings; sealed cartridge bearings generate 10 times the friction of unsealed cartridges; and grease lubrication generates six to seven times the friction of light oil. Also, slightly worn bearings and seals probably have lower energy losses than new bearings. In conclusion, clean and slightly worn cup and cone bearings with light-weight oil probably represent the most efficient transmission available today. Combined with a clean chain, chain ring, deraileur and rear cogs, drive train losses can be expected to be about 2–4% of the total energy input from the rider.

Rolling resistance

As bicycle tyres roll, the tread and casings (and enclosed tubes, if used) deform under load. A portion of this deformation is inelastic, and thus consumes energy. This energy loss is termed rolling resistance, and is represented by both static and dynamic components; the former does not vary with bicycle speed, while the latter does. Casing and tread construction, as well as tread design and tube construction, when used, affects rolling resistance. Thinner and more flexible casing designs have lower rolling resistance, as do light-weight natural rubber tubes and fine or slick tread patterns.

Rolling resistance is also affected by pavement roughness, wheel load, tyre pressure, tyre diameter, wheel diameter, tyre temperature, rear wheel propulsion and steering. Surface has a significant effect on rolling resistance, as do tyre pressure and wheel diameter. Note that slight increases in rolling resistance associated with smaller wheels and thinner tyres are offset by aerodynamic advantages. Higher temperatures reduce structural stiffness and increase tyre pressure, decreasing rolling resistance. Front-wheel rolling resistance increases with steering input, and rear energy losses occur when the bicycle is

accelerated, causing rear wheel propulsive torque and tread scrubbing. Practically speaking, rolling resistance can best be minimized using light-weight, flexible, ultra-high-pressure tyres with minimal tread on smooth concrete. Table 2.1 lists typical values for static rolling resistance coefficients (Crr_1 in the equation of motion). As shown, resistive forces created at the tyres are small but not insignificant. A dynamic coefficient of rolling resistance (Crr_2) of $0.05 \, \mathrm{N \cdot m \cdot s^{-1}}$ is recommended until more test results become available.

Power of climbing and descending

Bicycle manufacturers have spent considerable time and money on reducing the weight of bicycles. This effort has principally been motivated by the effects of gravity on cycling power. Gravity naturally causes power to increase dramatically during hill climbs, reducing efforts on descents. Unfortunately, the energy saved on downhills never offsets the added energy of climbing, due largely to aerodynamic

Table 2.1 Static rolling resistance coefficients (Crr_1) for common bicycle tyres. Resistance to bicycle motion is determined by multiplying the rider plus bicycle weight on each tyre by the coefficient shown divided by 100. Adapted from Kyle (1996).

Tyre type	Tyre size (mm)	Pressure (Pa)	On linoleum	On concrete	On asphalt
Tubular tyres					
Continental Olympic	686×19	6.89×10^5	0.19	0.17	0.22
Continental Olympic	610×19	6.89×10^5	0.26	0.23	0.27
Clement Colle Main	686×19	6.89×10^5	0.16		
Clement Colle Main	610×19	6.89×10^5	0.21		
Clement Colle Main	508×19	6.89×10^5	0.29		
Clincher tyres					
Specialized Turbo S	700×19	6.89×10^5	0.26		0.29
Specialized Turbo S, Kevlar wall/latex tube	700×19	6.89×10^5	0.23	0.27	
Specialized Turbo S, Kevlar wall/butyl tube	700×19	6.89×10^5	0.28		
Specialized Turbo S, Kevlar wall/polyurethane tube	700×19	6.89×10^5	0.29		
Specialized Turbo S, Kevlar wall/polyurethane liner	700×19	6.89×10^5	0.54		

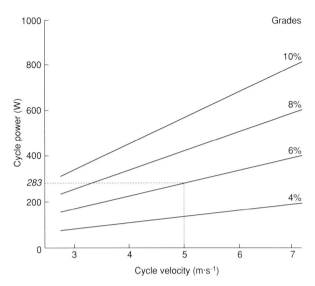

Fig. 2.19 Power required to climb for a 64 kg rider on an 8 kg bicycle for various conditions of speed and percentage grade. Power to overcome aerodynamic drag and rolling resistance are not included. Data can be scaled to heavier or lighter riders by multiplying the power determined on the graph by the ratio of the total rider plus bicycle weights (e.g. for a 90 kg rider plus bicycle system, power equals value on graph multiplied by 90/72).

effects, and thus hilly courses are slower than flat courses of the same length.

The equation of motion shows how bicycle power changes with grade. Fig. 2.19 shows power to climb (not including power to overcome aerodynamic drag and rolling resistance) as a function of bicycle velocity, grade and rider plus bicycle weight. Power for a 64 kg rider on an 8 kg bicycle to climb a 6% grade at 5 m · s⁻¹ (18 km · h⁻¹) equals 283 W. Given that maximum steady-state power outputs for world-class cyclists are in the 400−450 W range, it is easy to see from Fig. 2.18 why cycling velocities decrease rapidly as grades increase.

Inertial effects

Bicycles accelerate when average power produced by the rider exceeds the sum of the aerodynamic, rolling, grade and bearing resistances. The acceleration is directly proportional to the net force produced at the rear-wheel contact patch and inversely proportional to rider plus bicycle mass. Consequently, lighter

bicycles can be accelerated faster. An 80 kg rider plus bicycle system accelerating uniformly over 100 m in 10 s will accelerate at 2 m · s⁻¹. The same effort (propulsive force) applied to a rider and bicycle with an additional 1 kg (81 kg total) will result in the rider being approximately 1 m behind at the 100 m mark. Since normal races incorporate many decelerations and accelerations, lighter bicycles provide the racing cyclist with a slight advantage. Finally, during bicycle acceleration, both wheels are angularly accelerated, and their rotational inertias resist this acceleration. Light wheels with their mass concentrated closer to the hub are easier to accelerate than wheels with the mass closer to the rims.

Aerodynamics

At speeds above 11 m · s⁻¹ (40 km · h⁻¹), aerodynamic drag represents more than 80% of the total resistive drag on a cyclist and bicycle. Standard racing bicycles are responsible for approximately 35% of the total aerodynamic drag; the remainder is attributed to the rider's body. Streamlined time-trial bicycles may represent only 20% of the total aerodynamic drag. Nevertheless, both rider and bicycle create the vast majority of resistance to forward progression, and thus attention to managing and reducing aerodynamic drag from all sources is well rewarded (Fig. 2.20).

Bicycle frame

Perhaps the most striking characteristic of today's aerodynamic superbikes is the shape and configuration of the major frame structural elements. Round head tubes, down tubes, seat tubes and top tubes have been replaced by ovalized or airfoil sections with major to minor diameter ratios as high as 5 : 1 (i.e. they are five times longer than they are wide). Round spokes on non-disc wheels have also been replaced by ovalized aero spokes. The reasoning behind using airfoil sections for spokes and frame elements is understood by considering how air flows around these shapes. A round cylinder creates a turbulent wake with a trailing low-pressure region that generates high drag. The coefficient of drag (see the equation of motion) for such a cylinder is 1.2. An ovalized airfoil section in an air stream creates a smooth surface over which the air flows, without turbulence. The airfoil

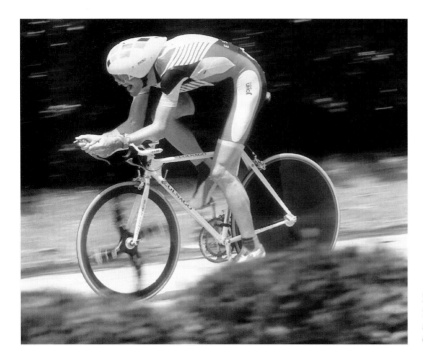

Fig. 2.20 Atlanta 1996: individual time trial. Abraham Olano (ESP) in an aerodynamic position, second. © Allsport / Pascal Rondeau.

can have one-tenth the drag of the cylinder given the same frontal area (C_d = 0.1 or less).

In addition to the shape of the individual frame elements, the arrangement of frame elements also affects air flow and drag. The air stream passing over a conventional double-diamond bicycle at a level just above the axles must pass across four frame elements: the fork, the down tube, the seat tube and the rear seat stays. A review of the common superbike frame arrangements (Fig. 2.21) shows that there are many ways to reduce the number of times the air stream passes over a frame element. Bicycle designers also strive to make air stream interactions with the frame as aerodynamically clean as possible, incorporating frame elements as narrow as structurally permissible with smooth transitions between adjacent elements.

An interesting feature of aerodynamic bicycles is the air stream interaction with the rider. Wind-tunnel tests have shown that some bicycles are very aerodynamic (have low drag) when tested as a riderless bicycle, but with a rider the bicycle performs comparatively worse. The reason appears to be that some frame arrangements cause obstruction of the flow

stream between the rider's legs at certain positions in the pedal cycle. Naturally this effect depends on the rider's leg muscular development and the arrangement of frame elements. Nevertheless, drag-producing interactions between riders and their supposedly aerodynamic bicycles should not be overlooked.

Bicycle components

Intelligent selection of bicycle components can significantly reduce aerodynamic drag. Table 2.2 lists the aerodynamic consequences of selecting specific bicycle components, in terms of their resulting drag reduction at 13.4 m · s^{-1} (48.4 km · h^{-1}). Many of these modifications are inexpensive to incorporate, produce time savings well within typical separations between competitors in international events, and have become standard features on today's superbikes. Incidentally, 0.1 N of drag is produced by placing roughly 0.1 m of a pencil perpendicularly into an air stream at 13.4 m · s^{-1} (48.4 km · h^{-1}). Many bicycle components, such as cables, water-bottle cages and seat rails, resemble pencil-like shapes.

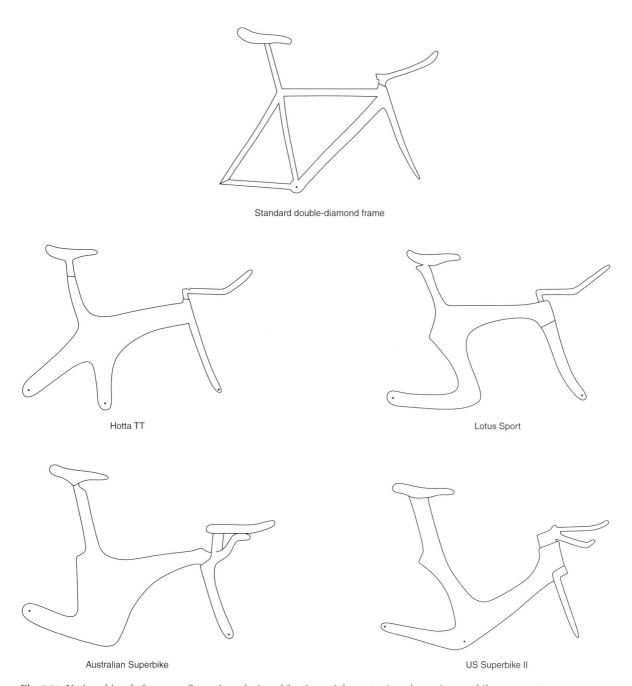

Standard double-diamond frame

Hotta TT

Lotus Sport

Australian Superbike

US Superbike II

Fig. 2.21 Various bicycle frame configurations designed for time-trial events. Aerodynamic superbikes attempt to (i) minimize the number of times the air stream crosses frame structural elements; (ii) limit drag-producing interactions between the air stream, the frame and the rider's legs; and (iii) incorporate smooth transitions between frame elements.

Table 2.2 Aerodynamic advantages of various bicycle components. Drag force shown for 13.4 m · s⁻¹ (48.4 km · h⁻¹) bicycle velocity. Adapted from Kyle (1995).

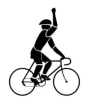

	Drag force (mN)
Cranks and sprockets	
Modified TA crank with 1 disc, 52T sprocket (reference)	+0
Same crank with normal 52T sprocket	+39
Standard Shimano crank with one 42T sprocket	+108
Standard Shimano crank with one 52T sprocket	+137
Standard Shimano crank with 52 and 42T sprockets	+206
Pedal systems	
Clipless pedals, Shimano/Look-type system (reference)	+0
Shimano pedals, toe clips and straps	+235
Campagnalo pedals, toe clips and straps	+235
Miscellaneous	
Aero shifters on down tube (reference)	+0
Normal down tube shifters, levers up	+78
Sheathed cable, perpendicular to air stream	+500 per metre
Bare cable, perpendicular to air stream	+155 per metre
Aero handlebars (airfoil sections), no drop bars	−755
Water bottle behind seat (compared to down tube)	−784
Aero water bottle and cage compared to standard	−127

Wheels

Carefully controlled tests in wind tunnels have exposed the aerodynamic advantages and disadvantages of bicycle wheels, in both head-wind (normal riding) and cross-wind conditions. Since a rider is responsible for providing the energy both to spin and propel the wheels (and bicycle) through the air, tests are usually performed by spinning the wheel at wind-tunnel air speed and measuring both the aerodynamic drag on the wheel and the power required to spin the wheel. The results of wind-tunnel testing have produced the following general conclusions.

1 Disc wheels or three-spoke composite wheels are superior to any spoked wheel, including 16 blade aero-spoked wheels with aero rims. Also, lens-shaped disc wheels (thicker at the hub than the rim) are superior to flat discs.

2 Significant drag reduction is achieved by using narrow 18 mm tyres.

3 Smaller-diameter wheels have lower aerodynamic drag than larger wheels.

4 Aero-bladed and oval spokes are dramatically superior to round spokes, and of course fewer spokes are better.

5 Flat rims create turbulent flow over their trailing edges that creates drag. Aero rims provide a trailing edge that reduces turbulence and thus drag.

6 The aerodynamic drag of disc wheels and three-spoke composite wheels decreases in mild cross winds due to aerodynamic lift.

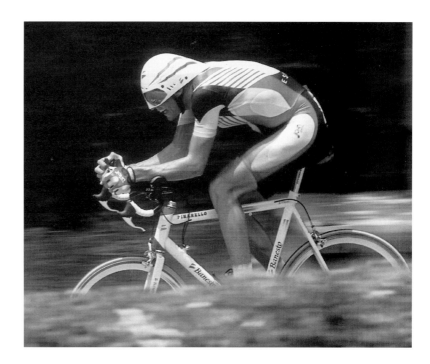

Fig. 2.22 Atlanta 1996. Miguel Indurain (ESP), first. © Allsport / Pascal Rondeau.

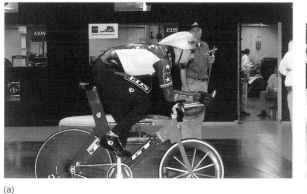

(a)

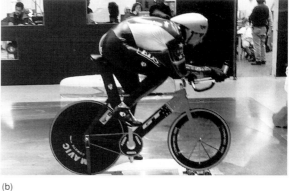

(b)

Fig. 2.23 A US national team rider in the General Motors wind tunnel in (a) a fatigued posture and (b) a stream-lined more forward position. At a constant effort, the difference between the two positions, calculated from the measured drag, would be 61.37 m and 3.91 s at the finish line.

Rider position effects

As previously stated, racing bicycles are responsible for roughly 20–35% of the total aerodynamic drag; the remainder is attributed to the rider's body. Experiments in wind tunnels and controlled tests using on-board power measurement devices have shown that a cyclist riding with a flat back, head lowered and forearms positioned parallel to the bicycle frame (on clip-on bars, for example) experiences dramatically less aerodynamic drag than a less stream-lined rider (Fig. 2.22).

A US national team rider is shown in Fig. 2.23 in the General Motors wind tunnel in two slightly different positions. In Fig. 2.23(a), the rider assumed what his coach described as his fatigued posture. His aerodynamic drag in this position, measured at a wind speed of 13.4 m · s^{-1} (48.4 km · h^{-1}) was 23.57 N. When

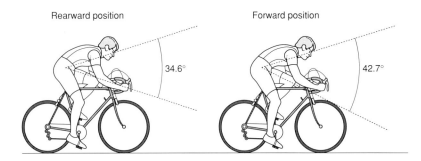

Rearward position   Forward position

34.6°   42.7°

Fig. 2.24 The aerodynamic position causes the hip to be more flexed through the top of the pedal stroke, often disturbing pedalling quality. By moving the saddle forward and slightly upward, the hip is opened up, interference between the legs and chest is less likely and the position resembles more normal cycling.

he lowered his head, extended his aerodynamic handlebars 0.02 m, and dropped his handlebar stem 0.02 m (Fig. 2.23b), his drag decreased to 22.28 N. The effect of this 1.29 N difference on a 4000 m individual time trial, at constant mechanical power output, was calculated to be 61.37 m or 3.91 s at the finish line! Many international events are decided by fractions of this difference.

Some riders have difficulty achieving the flat-back position. In particular, this position involves forward rotation of the pelvis, which tends to place the hip in greater flexion at the top of the pedal stroke. Increased hip flexion effectively lengthens the hip extensor muscles (gluteals and hamstrings), while shortening the hip flexor muscles (rectus femoris and iliopsoas) relative to their normal operating conditions. These changes in muscle-operating conditions compromise some riders' ability to pedal the bicycle effectively. The effect, observable with force-measuring pedals, is most noticeable in the upstroke and across the top of the pedal cycle.

The increased hip flexion created by the forward rotation of the pelvis, in conjunction with the forward position of the torso, can also cause interference problems between the thigh and chest. Cyclists with long tibia in relation to femur lengths, and/or large lower-torso girth, are particularly prone to this interference problem. To avoid compromising pedalling mechanics in favour of enhanced aerodynamic positioning, a solution is a slight forward and upward motion of the saddle. Such saddle motion effectively opens up the hip angle to better replicate the standard riding position (Fig. 2.24). This is the reason why triathletes and time-triallists often ride bicycles with steeper seat tubes.

The Union Cycliste Internationale (UCI) currently limits the fore–aft position of the saddle such that the

nose of the saddle is positioned at least 5 cm behind the bottom bracket spindle. This rule, which discourages extreme forward positioning on the bicycle, can be waived for anthropomorphic reasons.*

Regarding the fore–aft position of the arms, recent wind-tunnel and instrumented track testing has been revealing. Firstly, at the time of writing the most aerodynamic rider position is the 'superman' position, which places the rider's hands and arms stretched out in front of the body. Chris Boardman used the 'superman' position during his successful hour record attempt. This position has the effect of lowering surface area, and probably the coefficient of drag as well, by allowing riders to shrug their shoulders and place their head and torso somewhat in the wake (or draft position) behind the hands and arms. In late 1996, the UCI enacted bicycle restrictions to prevent cyclists from riding in the 'superman' position. Specifically, the furthest forward position of the handlebars was limited to 80 cm forward of the bottom bracket spindle. Interestingly, shorter riders and/or riders with short torsos can still achieve a superman-like position, or a reasonably effective facsimile of one, despite this 80 cm rule. New UCI restrictions, which were introduced in 1998, prohibit all cyclists from using the 'superman' position.

Research findings are largely inconclusive on whether to place the arms together or apart on aerodynamic handlebars. Anecdotal evidence suggests that a combination of factors may dictate whether the arms should be together or apart. With the arms

---

* Shorter riders have difficulty meeting the 5 cm UCI rule because it forces them to ride with exceptionally shallow seat tube angles. Short riders are thus often allowed to ride with their saddles in front of the 5 cm limit.

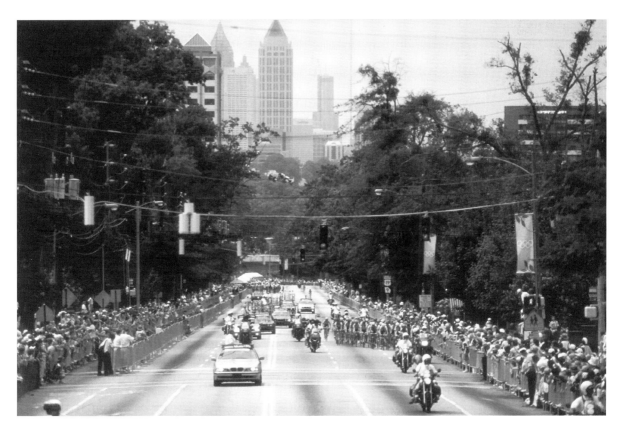

Fig. 2.25 Atlanta 1996: general view in the town. © Allsport / Nathan Bilow.

together, a large portion of the air stream is presumably directed around the rider's body. With the forearms separated, a significant portion of the air stream passes over the handlebars, beneath the rider's chest, between the legs and across the seat tube toward the rear wheel. The arms-together position may be more appropriate for the rider who has difficulty achieving a narrow and rounded position of the shoulders with the elbows and forearms apart, and/or rides a bicycle with a round seat tube and a non-aero-spoked rear wheel. In this case, the rider effectively directs a significant portion of the air stream around the body and away from the high-drag frame and rear wheel. Conversely, the latter position may be appropriate for the rider who can become

narrow through the shoulders even with the arms apart, and rides an aero bicycle with a rear disc wheel. Additional research should establish optimal combinations for riders and bicycles of various configurations.

Finally, significant changes in body position on the bicycle should be made slowly and incrementally, because firstly, the flat-back position places greater stress on the lower back and neck, and secondly, the aero position places more weight on the front wheel, and thus may compromise bicycle stability and handling. Training time should be devoted to experimenting with more forward positions in order to adapt to the modified skeletal loads and gain familiarity with alterations in bicycle handling.

Chapter 3

Testing methods in road cycling

Functional evaluations of the cyclist must take into account the athlete–bicycle combination. Thus, the following components must be considered: metabolics, biomechanics (transforming metabolic work into mechanical work) and aerodynamics (transforming mechanical work into speed). The interaction of these components determines the road cyclist's performance capacity.

Laboratory testing

The bicycle has been used for many years in the field of exercise physiology as a standard form of ergometry. The stationary bicycle whose front or back wheel is driven by the subject's pedalling typically offers resistance through a frictional band or by electromagnetic braking. The work load can quickly and easily be adjusted by changing the tension (and hence the frictional load) of the brake band or the electromagnetic load across a generator. Work is typically calculated from a scale reading which provides the frictional resistance or force and from a counter that records the number of times the wheel has turned, providing a calculation of distance: $D = 2\pi RN$ (Radius of wheel and Number of revolutions). The work performed by the rider is then calculated with knowledge of the force and the distance through which the force is applied. This piece of equipment, the stationary bicycle, is relatively inexpensive and greatly facilitates measurement of oxygen consumption, heart rate (HR) and various other physiological measurements needed in an exercise physiology setting. The disadvantages of this traditional form of ergometry, however, rest on the fact that the bike is rarely suited to the rider, the rider is generally unfamiliar with this type of exercise, and

it is well known that a maximum oxygen consumption value on the bicycle, in most individuals, will be lower than on the treadmill. Physiological efficiency is then typically calculated knowing the caloric equivalent through oxygen consumption and the amount of work done on the bicycle. Hence, the bicycle has a long history in providing a standard form of testing and evaluating performance and work done by subjects in studies that involve a variety of experimental conditions.

Recent interest in evaluating cycling mechanics, bicycle components and competitive cyclists themselves has generated a large number of new and innovative laboratory bicycle ergometers. These ergometers range from systems such as rollers that are designed to load each individual's personal bicycle to systems that involve standard road or track bicycles instrumented to measure handlebar loads, loads on the seat and interactive forces of the pedals, using systems described in Chapter 2. The primary criterion in the development of these systems is that they provide an environment familiar to the competitive cyclists that can incrementally load each rider, resulting in a valid evaluation of cycling performance. Typical measurements made under these conditions involve kinematic and kinetic analyses as well as an evaluation of leg muscle patterns during the pedalling cycle. A common form of cycle ergometer using standard road or track bicycles involves wind-load simulators, described later.

Despite recent advances in ergometer design intended to customize the frame and components to the individual rider, no laboratory situation can easily replicate the aerodynamic challenge to the rider. Consequently, while testing in the laboratory might accommodate geometric considerations, it is difficult to investigate aerodynamic demands. In light of this challenge, many laboratory teams interested in evaluating bicycle position, cycling mechanics and aerodynamic drag take riders to wind tunnels to evaluate their position on the bicycle. Following testing in such a complicated environment as a wind tunnel, many laboratory teams then instrument bicycles on the track to monitor crank speed, forces at the pedal and power output in the bicycle. This combination of monitoring performance in laboratory-controlled conditions and on the track or road

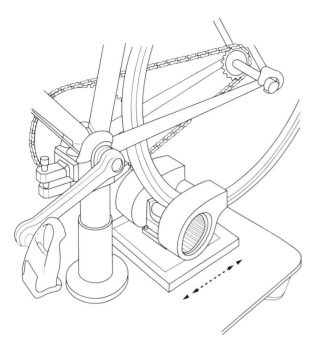

Fig. 3.1 Scheme of a wind-load bicycle simulator.

The subject's bicycle is mounted on a stand and equipped with a heavy (2.8 kg) rear wheel to increase the inertia of rotation (wheel circumference 2.12 m). The tubular tyre is inflated to a pressure of 810 kPa. The bicycle's rear wheel is in contact with a freely rotating axle with two fans attached to its extremities which impel air and create wind resistance. This roller with fans can be moved in a horizontal direction (see arrows on Fig. 3.1) with a micrometric screw and pressed against the tubular tyre so as to obtain variations in the rolling resistance. A standard crank set with a built-in power-measuring system (SRM training system, Ingenierbliro Schoberer, Jiilich-Welldorf, Germany) is mounted on the athlete's bicycle. This instrument is a torque transducer with 20 strain gauge strips applied between the axle of the bottom bracket set and the chain rings. Electric signals are digitized and are inductively and continuously transmitted from the moving power meter to a mini-computer fixed to the handlebars. At the same time, pedalling cadence is measured and transmitted to this minicomputer. The minicomputer calculates the data of the torque and angular velocity and averages the power of every complete revolution. It also measures the cyclist's HR with the help of a pulse trans-mitter and calculates the cycling speed by means of a magnet placed on a wheel. Data memorization is time based (e.g. 1 s).

For purposes of standardization, the pressure of the roller against the tyre is regulated to obtain a resist-ance of 100 W at 60 rpm, with a gear ratio of 52×15.

Warm-up procedure

Trained athletes must be well rested and perform an incremental warm-up for at least 30 min. The gear for the warm-up is selected after preliminary evaluations lasting 5 min, during which the subject, having chosen a certain gear, increases the cadence from 60 to 70 rpm (at a rate of 1 rpm every 30 s). If, during this preliminary test, HR increments exceed 8 beats · min[-1] per minute, the subject switches to a lower gear. The gear ratio that produces these HR increments in well-trained adult cyclists is generally a 52×15 or a 52×14; it is smaller in younger athletes, and even smaller in sedentary subjects. Once the gear has been selected, the athlete pedals for 30 s at 60 rpm. The

provides one of the best evaluation packages for monitoring cycling mechanics, aerodynamics and physiology. Once an aerodynamic position is established in a wind tunnel (and possibly patterns evaluated for lower-extremity musculature, force input to the crank or other interactive forces with the bicycle) these positions can be tested out on the track or road using on-board recorders designed to measure bicycle power output. This testing combination is now used by several laboratories throughout the world.

Aerobic power and the anaerobic threshold determination; the Conconi test on a wind-load simulator

Wind-load simulators allow one to reproduce, during testing, the increments of rolling resistance and air resistance typical of real cycling. The wind-load simulator shown in Fig. 3.1 also allows for tests in which athletes uses their own bicycle, and thus their habitual body position.

cadence is then increased by 1 rpm every 30 s until a cadence of 90–95 rpm is reached. After a 5 min recovery period of pedalling slowly, the warm-up is completed with variations at higher cadences (e.g. 110 rpm) of short duration (5–10 s), repeated 3–5 times. Following another 5 min recovery, the subject is ready to begin the test.

Test procedure

Using the gear selected for the warm-up, the athlete rides the bicycle in the racing position. The test is started at 60 rpm, and the cadence is increased by 1 rpm every 30 s until submaximal exercise intensity (EI) is reached. When the subject (or test assistant) becomes aware of physical signs of near-maximal effort, such as burning muscles or breathing difficulties, the uniform increases in cadence are substituted by a faster acceleration regulated by the test subject. In this phase, the increase in cadence occurs after progressively shorter time intervals (e.g. 10 s) and

continues up to the subject's maximal cadence (from 120 to 150 rpm), which is reached in 2–3 min.

Data analysis

The data collected during testing are analysed by a personal computer, and the EI/HR relationship is plotted in a graph form.

For the EI/HR relationship, the correlation coefficient (r) and slope (b) of the straight-line equations, obtained with the addition of each subsequent data point, are calculated. The point of passage from the linear phase of the EI/HR relationship to the curvilinear phase (the so-called deflection point) is identified as that above which the values of b begin to decrease (arrowed in Fig. 3.2). The detailed test procedure has been published in 1999 by the *Med. Sci. Sports Exerc* **Vol 31**, 1478–83.

The same procedure is used to analyse the EI/V_{O_2} relationship, when determined. Determining the EI/HR relationship provides information that is useful for

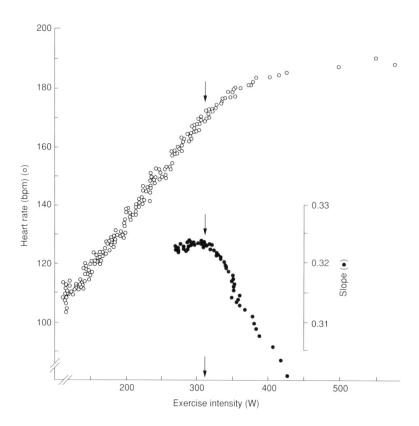

Fig. 3.2 Exercise intensity/heart rate relationship (○) during an incremental test on a wind-load simulator in a cyclist. The data points represent average of 5-second intervals. The slope values (●) of the straight-line equations calculated on the data points are also indicated. Arrows: deflection point.

evaluating the athlete and any changes brought about through training programmes. The most important of these are:

1 the point of deflection, that is, the point of passage from the linear to the curvilinear phase of the EI/HR relationship; this point coincides with the anaerobic threshold (AT). For practical purposes, the watts, HR and oxygen consumption (Vo_2, when available) at deflection should also be considered;

2 maximal heart rate and aerobic power (Vo_{2max}) of the subject under test;

3 the slope of the straight line describing the EI/HR and EI/Vo_2 relationship: the lower the slope of the straight line, the better the subject's cardiocirculatory functioning.

When, during the incremental test, respiratory gases are determined, AT can be determined by analysing the relationship between carbon dioxide output and oxygen uptake, following Wassermann's classic method. AT can also be determined by measuring blood lactate concentration at various exercise intensities (lactate concentration increases sharply above AT).

Evaluation of anaerobic lactacid power

Information on anaerobic lactacid power can be obtained from all-out tests carried out using the wind-load simulator and the athlete's bicycle as described above (Fig. 3.2). In all-out efforts, creatine phosphate is exhausted in 6–8 s. Therefore, in the first 6–8 s, work output can be attributed to the anaerobic alactacid mechanism, and from 10 to 20 s, to the full activation of the anaerobic lactacid mechanism. The average power generated between 10 and 20 s in an all-out 20 s test is therefore indicative of the anaerobic lactacid mechanism of the subject. In elite cyclists, it ranges from 650 to 950 W, with the highest values being found in sprinters. Subjects having great anaerobic lactacid power can reach lactate concentrations that are much higher than those of more aerobic subjects. Nevertheless, determination of blood lactate concentration in all-out tests does not provide accurate data on anaerobic lactacid power since lactate concentration can vary according to the muscular mass employed, the duration of the all-out effort, the rate of the subject's lactate removal mechanism and the kinetics of activation of the aerobic mechanism.

Determination of anaerobic lactacid endurance

There are no specific tests to measure anaerobic endurance (the maximal amount of work that can be performed with anaerobic lactacid adenosine triphosphate resynthesis). Information on anaerobic lactacid power can be obtained from all-out tests carried out using the wind-load simulator and the athlete's bicycle as described in Fig. 3.1 (p. 41). The total work carried out in these tests includes that performed with the anaerobic alactacid mechanism and with the aerobic mechanism, which is partially activated.

Non-laboratory methods

Outdoor tests, which can be carried out on a velodrome, on a straight flat road or on a climb, have the advantage of measuring the cyclist under real cycling conditions, taking into account a fundamental variable in cycling: the aerodynamics of the cyclist–bicycle combination.

Outdoor tests are seriously complicated, however, by the difficulty of standardizing the testing conditions due to:

1 variations in air resistance, because frictional air resistance increases relative to the square of the speed. In cycling, speeds are reached at which air resistance is considerable (e.g. at 60 km · h^{-1}, 90% of the total power output is used to overcome air resistance). Therefore, even small changes in air density (due to variations in humidity, temperature and atmospheric pressure) or the presence of wind will influence the cyclist's speed and EI and therefore the determination of the EI/HR relationship;

2 variations in rolling resistance, which depend on the different surfaces found on the velodrome and the road. Acceptable conditions for the functional evaluation of the cyclist are firstly, an indoor velodrome, because of lack of wind and controlled temperature and humidity; and secondly, a hill with a constant slope, where the slow speed renders negligible the influence of variations in air resistance.

Determination of the anaerobic threshold in an indoor velodrome

Determination of the AT through the EI (watts or speed)/HR relationship can be carried out on an indoor velodrome following the same procedure for warm-up, performance of the incremental test and data analysis as in the laboratory test.

In the incremental tests performed on the indoor velodrome, wide oscillations in speed have been observed; the cyclist's speed increases in the curves and decreases in the straight sections. Wide oscillations in the athlete's power are also present, often in phase opposition to speed (Fig. 3.3). These oscillations can easily be seen when data collection is frequent (e.g. five per second).

To explain this unforeseen observation, we must divide the athlete–bicycle combination schematically into two parts: firstly, the upper part (above the saddle), which includes the cyclist's head, trunk and upper limbs, and secondly, the lower part (from the saddle down), which includes the frame, wheels and the cyclist's lower limbs. In the straight sections of the velodrome, the upper part of the cyclist–bicycle combination proceeds at the same speed as the lower. In the curved sections, the athlete leans towards the centre of the bending radius, and the two parts advance simultaneously on two different semicircumferences and, therefore, at different speeds. For example, on a curve with a semicircumference of 70 m (bending radius 22.29 m), if we assume that the athlete's inclination results in a reduction in the radius of 1.2 m, his or her upper part will run on a semicircumference of 66.23 m. The two semicircumferences will be covered simultaneously but at different speeds: if the trunk travels at 50 km $\cdot$ h^{-1}, the wheels will travel at 52.874 km $\cdot$ h^{-1}. It must be kept in mind that the cyclist's speed is calculated at the wheels and thus using the larger semicircumference.

Each time the cyclist exits from a curved section, wheel speed decreases, and the speed of the lower and upper parts becomes the same again. The increases in speed in the curves are a function of the bending radius and the steepness of the curves and thus vary from velodrome to velodrome. The continuous oscillations in the cyclist's speed on the velodrome are accompanied by wide oscillations, often cyclical, in the cyclist's EI, with decreases in the curves and increases in the straight sections.

This discontinuity in physical effort renders the determination of the EI/HR relationship more difficult and less than optimal on a velodrome, given that the continuous oscillations in EI could cause early activation of the anaerobic mechanisms. The EI/HR

relationship can, however, be determined on an indoor velodrome and can be added to that obtained on a wind-load simulator when considering the average values for the 30 s fractions into which the test is subdivided.

In 14 cyclists riding on an indoor velodrome at an average power output of 400 W, the speed ranged from 42.7 to 46.2 km/h^{-1}. For athlete number 15 who used three different bicycles (solid bars), the speed at 400 W ranged from 42.7 to 46.9 km/h^{-1} (Fig. 3.4).

These observations demonstrate that indoor velodrome tests provide information on the aerodynamics of the cyclist–bicycle combination and show that speed is not an absolute measure of the cyclist's EI, which is better expressed in watts, even in indoor velodrome testing.

Determination of the anaerobic threshold on a hillclimb

Determination of the EI/HR relationship can be carried out on a hillclimb following the same procedure for the laboratory test. The selection of the hill is fundamental: it should have a constant slope of more than 8% (in order to exclude speeds at which variations in aerodynamics can invalidate the collected data) and no switchbacks. Climbing ability can also be measured on the road and expressed in terms of metres of altitude change per hour (vertical ascending rate). This can be accomplished by doing a time trial on a climb for which the exact change in altitude is known. During stage races on long climbs, professional cyclists have been recorded to attain ascending rates of 1800 m $\cdot$ h^{-1}.

Aside from changes due to training, modifications in ascending rate are closely related to the weight of the cyclist–bicycle combination.

Testing for aerobic endurance in road cycling

The road cyclist is expected to race, and therefore train, for several consecutive hours. When adequately trained for endurance, the athlete's aerobic and anaerobic power remain unaltered during the entire length of the effort. By contrast, when aerobic endurance training is insufficient, aerobic and anaerobic power diminish progressively. The decrease in aerobic power during a prolonged effort is due

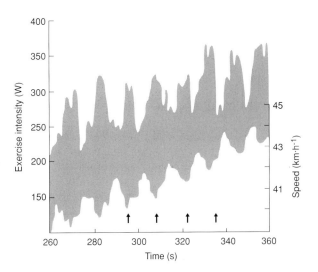

Fig. 3.3 Trends over time of exercise intensity (EI) and speed (S) in an incremental test performed on an indoor velodrome. Cyclical oscillations of EI and S, in phase opposition, are observed twice per lap. The higher S are reached in the curved sections of the tract, the higher EI in the straightaway sections. The four arrows indicate the beginning of the curved sections for two consecutive laps. The upper grey portion of the graph represents EI, the lower white portion S (Alfieri N. and Conconi F., unpublished observations).

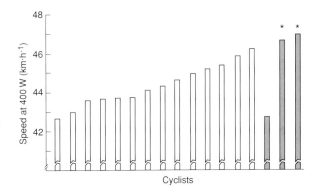

Fig. 3.4 Speed values corresponding to an exercise intensity of 400 W obtained on an indoor velodrome by 14 professional cyclists (open bars) and by one cyclist (solid bars) using a standard racing and two time-trial (*) bicycles (Alfieri N. and Conconi F., unpublished observations).

primarily to a drop in glycogen reserves, which also brings about a reduction in anaerobic lactacid power. It is possible to monitor the endurance of a road cyclist by performing repeated functional evaluations, as follows (see also training for aerobic endurance, Chapter 4).

1 Determination of the EI/HR relationship in incremental tests on a wind-load simulator, interrupting the test before the final acceleration. The athlete performs this determination three times during a long training session. In an athlete who is not adequately trained for endurance, the EI/HR relationship will move towards the left when plotted on a graph.

2 Determination of the power produced in an all-out 10 s test, performed at the end of each of the three determinations described in point 1. The maximum and average wattage obtained will not decrease substantially in the endurance-trained athlete.

3 Performance, during a long training session, of tests at race pace on an 8–10 km hillclimb with a slope of more than 8%, recording HR and measuring ascending rate. The endurance-trained athlete will maintain almost constant values in the various tests. These tests cannot usually be carried out on a flat road because variations in environmental conditions would invalidate the results.

4 The exhaustion of glycogen reserves that can be observed in athletes lacking sufficient endurance training at the end of long training sessions can be confirmed by the presence of acetone in the urine. This test can easily be performed using commercially available sticks.

Chapter 4

Training the physiological characteristics employed in road cycling

Unlike sports characterized by the prevalent use of only one of the three mechanisms of adenosine triphosphate resynthesis (e.g. high jump, anaerobic alactacid; 400 m run, anaerobic lactacid; marathon, aerobic mechanism), road cycling involves their combined use, in percentages that vary with the course and type of race (whether mass start or individual time trial). Consequently, all three mechanisms must be considered when testing and training the cyclist.

The road cyclist must possess an aerobic mechanism that is well developed in both power and endurance. Aerobic power is required in several phases of road cycling, such as breakaways, climbing and time trials. In addition, in the anaerobic phases of competition, rapid recovery of creatine phosphate stores and quick removal of lactate (which depend on the aerobic mechanism) are necessary. Aerobic endurance, while necessary in all types of road races, is especially important in stage racing.

The anaerobic mechanisms come into play in many shorter but critical phases of road cycling, such as closing gaps, short climbs at all-out speed, sprints out of corners or curves and finishing sprints.

The physical effort of the road cyclist varies not only with the competitive level of the race, which depends on the athletes involved, but also with the course (extremely variable) and with the atmospheric conditions. In addition to the energy-producing mechanisms required for muscular contraction, there are the important functions of thermoregulation, intestinal absorption and the capacity to restore glycogen reserves (as in stage racing), to cite but a few examples. Therefore, these functions must also be trained.

The different types of training that bring about improvements in power and endurance of the various forms of energy metabolism are described separately here. Naturally, these monothematic activities must be appropriately mixed during each training session and in the general training programme, taking into consideration the individual cyclist's characteristics and the types of races in which he or she will compete.

Training the aerobic mechanism

Development of the aerobic mechanisms of adenosine triphosphate production is indispensable for road cyclists and is the foundation for every training programme. It is easy to improve this mechanism despite the fact that important genetically determined differences exist in the individual's response to training. Prolonged suspension of training results in rapid regression.

Training for aerobic power

Training to improve aerobic power stimulates the development of both oxygen transport to the tissues (and thus the cardiocirculatory system) and aerobic fuel breakdown (and thus the mitochondria). Aerobic training usually stimulates both the central (cardiocirculatory) and peripheral (neuromuscular) components of aerobic metabolism. Training at high altitude principally develops the cardiocirculatory components.

Warm-up

Each training session for the road cyclist should be preceded by an adequate warm-up, during which the various mechanisms of energy production are progressively activated. The aerobic mechanism is activated by a slow progression (30 min or more) with the exercise intensity (EI) ranging from low to submaximal. Such a progression can be performed using the same moderate gear and gradually increasing the cadence. The fact that the warm-up is gradual prevents activation of the lactacid mechanism and activates both the cardiocirculatory and muscular phases of the aerobic mechanism. The athlete's preparation for the training session can be completed with several rapid accelerations of brief duration (5 s) that serve to activate the anaerobic mechanisms and the neuroendocrine system that controls them.

Training intensity

Theoretically, an improvement in any biological function can be attained through intense use of that function. Aerobic power can be improved by training that stimulates the maximal activation of the aerobic metabolism (training at Vo_{2max}). A second requirement for improving a certain function is that its employment should be sufficiently prolonged. This is impossible, however, for efforts at Vo_{2max}: such types of training are limited by the contemporaneous activation of anaerobic glycolysis and consequent lactate accumulation.

For this reason, training for aerobic power is performed at intensities lower than that at which the anaerobic lactacid mechanism is activated, that is, below the anaerobic threshold (AT). At these lower intensities, the training stimulus can be effected for much longer (when properly divided up) than is permitted by sessions at Vo_{2max} (a few minutes).

Planning for aerobic power training is made easier by identifying the AT and the corresponding heart rate (HR).

Experienced athletes are able to feel lactate accumulation in their muscles and thus identify subjectively the EI at which they should perform prolonged aerobic exercise.

During aerobic power training sessions, the athlete progressively attains the preselected submaximal EI and maintains it for several minutes. This type of interval work-out can be carried out either on the flat or on a hillclimb and is repeated several times; between the various intervals a recovery period of mild intensity is inserted. As training advances, the number and length of the work-outs can be increased. With time, the athlete is able to carry out prolonged intervals at an EI that coincides with the AT; he or she can even surpass this intensity during the final minutes of each interval. The EI should be adapted to variations in AT, which should ideally be checked regularly (every 2–3 weeks during the initial phases of training).

Training frequency

Submaximal exercise below AT, although less wearing than that which produces lactate, is a demanding effort and requires a recovery time appropriate to the assimilation capacity of the athlete in question. Information about the athlete's recovery can be obtained by testing his or her cardiocirculatory adaptation to incremental exercise: in the days immediately following work-outs, this response may be slower than usual, and the cyclist may fail to reach maximal HR (signs that may also occur with overtraining). These cardiocirculatory signs, in addition to the athlete's subjective feelings, can be used to establish the frequency of submaximal training. Considerable variations exist in the individual's recovery capacity from aerobic power training; however, in general, this type of work-out can be repeated every 3 days.

Training duration

It is advisable for cyclists who are not used to this type of training to begin with several work-outs lasting a few minutes each (e.g. three of 5 min). Well-trained cyclists, once they have reached their predetermined EI, maintain it for 15–20 min. In any case, recovery times should be similar to the interval times. Well-trained cyclists can do up to 2 h in 1 day of submaximal aerobic training, divided into shorter sessions.

Training for specific situations

Pedalling on the flat differs from hillclimbing in terms of, among other things, cadence, position in the saddle and the muscle groups employed. Even the cardiocirculatory involvement is different: in particular, the HR at AT is higher (usually by 3–5 beats · min⁻¹) in climbing than on the flat. The road cyclist must specifically train for riding under both conditions, performing the appropriate repeated aerobic work-outs, even during the same training session.

Training-induced changes

Aerobic power training brings about a series of structural and functional changes related to the reception and transport of *oxygen* (O_2) from the lungs to the muscles (respiratory exchange, cardiac function and muscular vascularization) and to the release and muscular utilization of O_2 (myoglobin, mitochondria and mitochondrial enzymes). These adaptations are evident in functional tests: Vo_{2max} increases slightly, AT increases considerably and the EI/Vo_2 and EI/HR relationships improve (the latter values shift to the right when plotted on a graph, so that every HR corresponds to a higher EI). At the same time, there is a reduction in resting HR, HR_{max} and HR corresponding to AT. As a consequence, the athlete's race pace (time-trial speed) will increase.

Training for aerobic endurance

It is well known that aerobic endurance is closely related to the capacity to perform intense muscular work while preserving glycogen reserves, thanks to the use of fuel mixtures rich in fatty acids. Therefore, training for aerobic endurance must improve not the muscular utilization of O_2, but rather the mixing of the two fuels, fatty acids and glycogen.

On this subject, it is important to remember that low-intensity exercise is primarily sustained by the combustion of fuel mixtures rich in fatty acids, while submaximal and maximal exercise requires mixtures rich in glucose. Medium-intensity exercise is sustained by the oxidation of both combustibles; medium and medium-high intensities, if carried out for a sufficiently long time, serve to orient the muscles towards the use of higher percentages of fatty acids, with a proportional reduction in glycogen consumption and thus an increase in endurance.

Training intensity, frequency and duration

Prolonged exercise at an intensity that is 15–20% below the AT has been shown to be efficacious in improving aerobic endurance. It is easy to recuperate from this type of training, so it can be performed every other day. Restoring glycogen reserves is fundamental to good recovery and should be done both during and after training (Chapter 5). Aerobic endurance training most resembles traditional training for cyclists (long and slow), although its intensity is higher than has been used in the past. This type of training can last from only 30 min in the initial phases of preparation

to 3 h or more (even if divided into shorter segments) in more advanced training phases. Aerobic endurance training is practised both on the flat and on long climbs as preparation for stage races. Distance training can be included in the longer training sessions (up to 7 h) that road cyclists sometimes practise twice a week, more often in a group than alone. It should be noted, however, that training for aerobic power and endurance should not be carried out while being 'pulled' by another cyclist: the speed may be right, but the cardiocirculatory and metabolic effort will be lower.

Training-induced changes

As endurance training progresses, and as the relative use of fatty acids increases with consequent sparing of glycogen, the EI/HR relationship is stabilized and there is a progressive reduction in the drifting-up of HR during prolonged submaximal exercise; this is a sign of developing endurance.

Monitoring aerobic training (Fig. 4.1)

An athlete can check whether his EI is was predetermined for the training session by using, during the work-out, the following indicators, singly or together:
1 subjective sensations: these are reliable in expert athletes;
2 HR, with an HR monitor;
3 pedalling cadence, speed and metres of altitude change per hour (ascending rate) in climbing;
4 power output in watts, using a commercially available power meter.

Subjective sensations are important, and the athlete with time learns to employ them. HR is a reliable indicator, although a drift towards higher values can be observed toward the end of the training session, especially in athletes who are still completing their endurance training. HR drifts can also be caused by variations in external conditions (wind, climbs, increased rolling resistance) that may activate the anaerobic mechanisms of the cyclist, who often concentrates more on speed than on EI. Measurement of power output (in watts) during training allows the athlete to control EI, thereby excluding the influence of external factors.

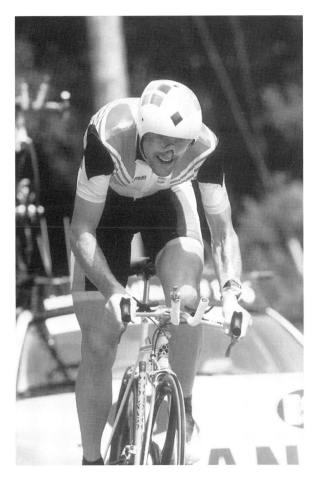

Fig. 4.1 Atlanta 1996: individual time trial. Abraham Olano (ESP), second. © Allsport / Nathan Bilow.

Training the anaerobic mechanism

Training for anaerobic power

Anaerobic power depends, in large part, on the percentage of fast-twitch fibres (genetically determined) and their recruitment, and on the consequent muscle metabolic characteristics of the athlete. Anaerobic power is much less responsive to training than is aerobic power. In fact, it is difficult to make a sprinter out of a 'slow' cyclist. The opposite can occur, however: a sprinter's top speed can be reduced if they practise aerobic training.

Often the road cyclist carries out anaerobic training through racing. Road racing requires frequent changes in EI and forces the cyclist to employ – and therefore develop – the anaerobic mechanisms. During winter training, only those road cyclists who intend to present themselves in top condition at the early-season races include anaerobic work-outs in their training programmes. Types of training that stimulate the development of anaerobic power are as follow.

1 Anaerobic alactacid power: maximal speed variations of 7–8 s, repeated up to 10 times, with a recovery of 2 min between variations. Up to three series of repetitions can be performed in each training session, with pauses lasting a few minutes between the series. They can be carried out on the flat or on climbs, starting at low EI, when good creatine phosphate reserves are available. Such series are inserted in the training programme beginning 30–40 days before the start of the racing season. They bring about a modest lactate accumulation and thus can be performed every day.

2 Anaerobic lactacid power: maximal speed variations of 30 s, repeated 3–5 times, with a 5 min recovery between each repetition. In a training session, 2–3 series of repetitions care be performed, with rest periods at low EI of 20 min between series. They can be carried out on the flat or on climbs, starting at exercise intensities near the AT. This avoids adding to the lactate accumulated during each speed variation, which is what would happen if starting from a low speed (O_2 debt). To facilitate the removal of lactate accumulated during each series, this training calls for ample rest periods and medium EI (e.g. 20% below AT) during the recovery periods. These workouts bring about a relatively high lactate concentration (muscular and blood) and thus can be carried out no more than three times a week; they are incorporated into the training programme beginning 30–40 days before the start of the racing season.

Training-induced changes

This type of training primarily causes muscular changes. In particular, it increases the concentrations of the enzymes for glycolysis and phosphocreatine kinase, as well as the speed of anaerobic glucose breakdown and the related anaerobic synthesis of adenosine triphosphate. In addition, the intermediate fibres specialize, in that they lose mitochondria and acquire glycolytic capacity. Although not ascertained, there are probably functional changes in the motor nerves of the muscular groups employed in this training and in the neuroendocrine system in general.

Training for anaerobic endurance

Road racing frequently requires prolonged lactacid work. Cyclists who possess well-developed anaerobic endurance have an advantage in those crucial phases of a race that require a maximal effort for several minutes, such as initiating or going with a breakaway, chasing down a small group of leaders or having the power necessary to make a strong effort at the finish (see finisseurs p. 17).

Training intensity, frequency and duration

This calls for training sessions similar to those used to develop anaerobic lactacid power, but of longer duration and with shorter recovery periods. The purpose of this type of training is to accumulate great quantities of lactate, thereby stimulating the anaerobic breakdown of glucose and the capacity to withstand high lactate concentrations. An example would be to perform variations of 60 s, at high EI, repeated 3–5 times, with a 3 min recovery between each variation. Recovery time can gradually be reduced to 2 min.

Training-induced changes

The increased capacity to withstand great quantities of accumulated lactate, possibly obtained by this training, could depend on improved efficiency of the buffering system in the individual's muscles. To date, not much is known about this buffering system. Improvements may also depend on an acceleration in lactate diffusion in the extracellular spaces and in the blood, lactate removal from the blood by the liver and heart, and lactate reuse by the muscles (immediately or in the recovery phase).

Specialized training for road cycling

1 Training of short duration at very high cadence. This consists of spinning low gears at a very high cadence (more than 150 rpm); in this way the cyclist becomes accustomed to the sudden variations in cadence encountered in many phases of racing. The duration of these bouts of maximal cadence may be 7–8 s, with up to 10 repetitions and a 2 min recovery between variations.

2 Training of long duration at high cadence. Traditionally used at the beginning of winter training, these work-outs are carried out using low gears at 100–110 rpm and can last up to 3 h. This form of training is intended to improve neuromuscular coordination.

3 Training at low cadence and high resistance. Carried out on a climb, this training consists of using high gears at a low cadence (even less than 40 rpm). Each work-out lasts 1–3 min, with a similar recovery time; work-outs can be repeated 3–6 times in a training session. This form of training is intended to improve muscular strength.

4 Muscular strengthening in the gymnasium. The road cyclist traditionally works out in the gym only at the beginning of winter training, for that short period in which training on the road is reduced to a few hours a week. The selected work-outs are performed at low intensity and high frequency. These work-outs are usually abandoned in January, when the greater number of hours on the road limits the time for other activities. Many cyclists now practise regular stretching exercises for specific muscles throughout the year.

A winter training schedule

An example of a training programme for a road cyclist who wants to be competitive beginning with the first races in February is given below.

November

Training calls for maintenance of the cardiocirculatory fitness developed during the previous season, with aerobic work-outs on the racing bike and also mountain biking, cycle-cross, running, swimming, cross-country skiing and roller- or ice-skating if the athlete has these abilities. The work-out intensity is that suggested for developing aerobic power and should reach the AT, but that level should only be maintained briefly. Training sessions should total 2–3 h a day, growing longer gradually (up to 3 h by the end of the month). Cycling sessions with a fixed gear should be included twice a week, and work-outs in the gym should be carried out every day.

December

Training for aerobic power and aerobic endurance should begin and progressively increase. Special sessions at low cadence and high resistance as well as at high cadence should be inserted twice a week (see above). Cycling with a fixed gear and work-outs in the gym should be continued. Non-specific aerobic exercise is discontinued. Training sessions should average 3–4 h a day, growing gradually longer (up to 4 h by the end of the month).

January

To the aerobic training sessions (in extension) are added the anaerobic ones, with the cadences, intensities and recovery times indicated in the section on training for anaerobic endurance (see above and Table 4.1).

The types of training indicated were explained earlier in this chapter. Medium intensity indicates an EI 20% below the AT. The long aerobic work-out of day 1, performed at medium intensity, if accompanied by nourishment that allows for reintegration of glycogen stores, is easy to recuperate from and permits the hard anaerobic endurance work-out of day 2. Days 3 and 4 call for training at medium intensity that enables recuperation from the anaerobic work-out of

day 2, accompanied by specific cadence and strength exercises. By day 5 the athlete is ready for the fatiguing aerobic power work-out, which requires a day of recuperation at medium intensity (day 6), preceding a day dedicated to anaerobic power (day 7). The cycle begins again with aerobic endurance training.

Tapering for road cycling

In contrast to athletes from other sports, the road cyclist does not practise tapering, that is, training at the usual EI but with a progressive reduction in duration for the 7–10 days before a race. The racing schedule (often two or more races a week) renders classic tapering impossible. In general, the athlete reduces training only for the day before a race.

Maintenance training during the racing season

During the racing season, which currently lasts 9 months from February through to October, the road cyclist has only brief non-racing periods (2–3 weeks at most). During these periods, in which it is best to recuperate, less demanding training should be carried out, primarily to mantain aerobic power and endurance.

Short-stage races for the major stage races

Long-stage races require a competitive effort that is repeated for many consecutive days and, therefore, need the development of special characteristics, in particular overnight recovery (including restoration of glycogen stores) and good performance on long climbs, which are generally not found in 1-day races. Since these situations are difficult to reproduce in training, preparation for the major stage races is completed by participating in stage races that last 5–6 days.

Recovery as a crucial part of training

Road cycling is a very demanding sport. Even train-ing for road cycling involves demanding exercise in terms of both length and intensity. It is important that hard work-outs, such as those to develop lactacid endurance, be followed by adequate recovery before

Table 4.1 A weekly training plan for the end of January.

Day	Type of training
1	Aerobic endurance (6 h)
2	Anaerobic endurance (3 h)
3	Medium-intensity and high-cadence–low-resistance exercise (3 h)
4	Medium-intensity and low-cadence–high-resistance exercise (3 h)
5	Aerobic power (5 h)
6	Medium-intensity exercise (3 h)
7	Anaerobic power (4 h)

Times given in parentheses indicate total training time, including warm-up and recovery periods.

carrying out another hard workout. Lack of recovery or incomplete recovery can be recognized by both subjective and objective signs. The athlete becomes aware of incomplete recovery mainly through muscular sensations. Among the easily identifiable objective signs are those connected with HR: it is lower than normal at various EIs and, in submaximal and maximal tests, the usual HRs are not reached (they are lower by as much as 10 bpm). The athlete struggles to perform these tests. When such conditions are found (signs can be seen even in the warm-up phase) it is best not to insist on the planned workout but rather to allow for adequate recovery. Insufficient recovery could lead to overtraining. In conclusion: begin training again when you are no longer tired.

Training for specific situations in road cycling

Time trialling

Good time-trial performance is important to success in stage racing. Recently, the winners of major stage races have built their success more on time trialling than on climbing ability (Fig. 4.2).

In a time trial lasting about 1 h, the athlete can maintain a medium EI corresponding to the AT. Thus, training for aerobic power and endurance, which the road cyclist does habitually, is the essential factor. Experienced endurance athletes are able to pace themselves and thus consume an optimal mixture of fatty acids and glycogen. This mixture allows them to burn the maximal amount of glycogen possible without depleting glycogen reserves before the end of the race. In a time trial, the cyclist can maintain a constant EI only theoretically: variations in environmental conditions can bring about an increase in speed, as compared to EI (e.g. with a tail wind or on a descent), but can also reduce speed (e.g. with a head wind, rough surface or on an ascent) so that the athlete is forced to deliver more power and to activate anaerobic mechanisms. Thus, the time triallist must also train and have available good anaerobic mechanisms. In training, the time triallist must become accustomed to changing position on the bike slightly (e.g. moving forward on the saddle), thereby modifying the muscular effort and allowing the muscles to recuperate from the effort.

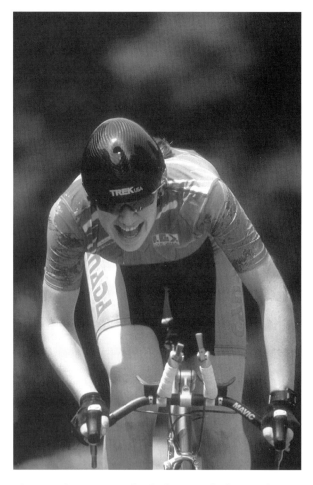

Fig. 4.2 Atlanta 1996: individual time trial. Clara Hughes (CAN), third. © Allsport / Nathan Bilow.

In preparing for time trials, particular attention is dedicated to the cyclist's position and aerodynamics; this is fundamental to obtaining good results.

Climbing

The action in climbing is different from that on the flat in terms of position in the saddle, muscles employed, cadence and force applied to the pedals. Also different is the action required in 1 day races on short, steep climbs (taken at speed, with relatively big gears, high applied force and large use of anaerobic mechanisms) from that required in stage races with long climbs taken with lower gears, at a more constant speed and using aerobic mechanisms almost exclusively. In addition to climbing in the saddle, which is typical of time triallists and 1-h racers, there is the alternating sitting–standing technique with accelerations which is typical of climbers. The obvious conclusion is that, for the various types and styles of climbing, specific training is required. In particular, preparation for 1-day races calls for anaerobic power and lactacid endurance work-outs on short, steep climbs, while preparation for stage races calls for aerobic power and endurance work-outs on long climbs.

Altitude training

Training at high altitude, which is practised more by athletes from other aerobic disciplines (e.g. running) than by road cyclists, consists of carrying out part of the training at 1800–3500 m above sea level. Sometimes the athlete spends periods at various altitudes, e.g. living at 3700 m and training at 1800 m above sea level (personal experience from Moser's hour record attempts in Mexico City). The length of stay at high altitude is usually 20–40 days. Following acclimatization of about 5 days (which varies with altitude and the individual's characteristics), when high-intensity exercise is avoided, the athlete resumes training.

The intensity of the various types of work-outs is established taking into account the physiological changes induced by high altitude and by the consequent reduced O_2 tension, which is evaluated with the usual laboratory and field tests.

Training-induced changes

The reduced O_2 availability at high altitude stimulates the mechanisms of O_2 transport from the lungs to the tissues due to an increase in the production of red blood cells, which gradually occurs during a 20–40 day stay at high altitude. The opposite result is obtained at the muscular level. The reduced O_2 availability permits aerobic exercise at a lower intensity than is possible at sea level, with consequent reduction in the mitochondrial functions and the muscular capacity to perform aerobic exercise; Vo_{2max} can be reduced after a 30 day stay at high altitude. The equilibrium between O_2 transport and its muscular utilization can be re-established at sea level through aerobic work-outs that stimulate the redevelopment of the mitochondrial functions. Such work-outs must be continued for 2–3 weeks in order to reap the benefits of the period spent at high altitude (personal observations).

Chapter 5

Nutrition for road cyclists

Introduction

Energy is the key to life. Any biological system depends on the availability of energy for building-up and metabolic processes. In humans, all energy is obtained from the combustion of energy containing nutrients, of which fat and carbohydrate (CHO) are of great importance. The energy expenditure of a sedentary adult with a body weight of 60–75 kg, whether male or female, is approximately 8.4–11.8 MJ (2000–2800 kcal) per day. Smaller, lighter individuals require less energy while heavier people who are physically active may require >12.6 MJ (3000 kcal) per day. Sports activity may increase daily energy expenditure by 2100 to over 4200 kJ (500–1000 kcal) per hour. The intensity as well as the duration of exercise are important in this respect. For example, a 200 m cycle sprint may cost only a few joules. The very short time during which such a highly intense performance is executed leads to only a slight increase in total daily energy expenditure. In contrast, endurance activities such as a 100 km cycling event or extended events such as the Tour de France will increase total daily energy requirements significantly. For example, the mean daily energetic cost of cyclists in the Tour de France was calculated to be ±27.3 MJ (6500 kcal) per day (for 21 days) with daily peaks up to >33 MJ (8000 kcal) when cycling in the Alps. Without doubt sufficient nutrients must be available as fuel. In the first part of this chapter we concentrate on different fuels in the body and their efficiency in supplying energy for muscular work. In the second part we focus on specific nutrient and non-nutritive food substances and their possible effects on performance.

Engines and fuels

The above-mentioned examples of energy expenditure show that exercise may lead to selective utilization of fuels available in the body. Sprinting requires only a relatively small amount of energy, but the rate at which this energy must be made available is extremely high. Thus, for sprinting, a type of fuel with rapid energy transfer characteristics is required. On the other hand, long-distance cycling requires a lower rate of energy production, but the large energy expenditure requires a large fuel supply. Human muscles are perfectly organized in this respect. For sprinting exercise, fast-twitch muscle fibres are activated by the nervous system. These fibres have a high capacity to perform anaerobic work and use exclusively fuel stores for energy production which allow for a high rate of energy transfer, i.e. creatine phosphate (CrP) and CHO. During endurance cycling, the nervous system primarily recruits slow-twitch muscle fibres. These fibres contract less rapidly, produce a lower peak power output, have a high resistance against fatigue and primarily use fat and CHO as fuel. Thus, the body selects both specific muscle fibres and specific fuels, depending on the intensity of the cycling event.

From an energy point of view, the maximum rate of energy transfer resulting from the breakdown of fuels within the muscle has been calculated (Table 5.1).

By far the highest energy production rate results from the breakdown of adenosine triphosphate (ATP) to adenosine diphosphate (ADP) and from CrP to creatine. The breakdown product, ADP, is a strong

Table 5.1 Maximum energy transfer (mmol ATP · g^{-1} muscle tissue · s^{-1}) from the conversion of different fuels in energy-reduced substrates. Reproduced with permission.

Fuel	End-product	Energy transfer index
Adenosine triphosphate, creatine phosphate	Adenosine diphosphate	2–3
Carbohydrate	Lactate	1.00
Carbohydrate	$CO_2 + H_2O$	0.50
Fat	$CO_2 + H_2O$	0.24

stimulator of glycolysis: CHO will be broken down at an increasing rate when ADP is high and the energy liberated will be used to regenerate ATP from ADP. The rate of energy transfer from the combustion of CHO, however, is slower than that from ATP and CrP. This results in a decreased rate of energy transfer, which causes a lower power output as soon as CHO becomes the dominant fuel. The consequence for practice is clear: power output and cycling speed in middle-distance events, such as the 1000 m time trial, are lower than in sprinting.

Fat is the 'slowest' fuel. This means that the rate of resynthesisis of ATP, when using fat as the main fuel, is even slower than when CHO is primarily used. From Table 5.1 we see that energy flow from fat, when broken down aerobically, is only one-half of that of CHO. It could be suggested that performance capacity should drop to 50% of maximum when CHO is depleted. Indeed, it has been observed that endurance performance capacity drops to about 40–50% of maximum when CHO availability becomes marginal and fat supplies most of the energy. However, the body never exclusively uses fat as fuel. For the aerobic oxidation of fat within the citric acid cycle, the muscle needs substrates to keep this cycle active at a high rate. These substrates, called citric acid cycle intermediates, to an large extent come from glycolysis. Thus, fat oxidation is not possible if pyruvate from CHO breakdown is not available. Therefore, when CHO (glycogen) depletion takes place, the body is increasingly activated to synthesize glucose from precursors such as lactate, glycerol and amino acids to cover the minimum of needs (Fig. 5.1). In particular, endurance-trained cyclists who frequently experience phases of limited CHO availability have improved gluconeogenic capacity.

From these data it can be concluded that there are three major fuels for the production of energy needed for muscular work: (i) a relatively small energy-rich phosphate pool; (ii) CHO; and (iii) fat.

In summary:

1 Muscle fibre-type recruitment and accompanying fuel selection depend on the intensity and duration of the exercise.

2 High-intensity exercise requires CrP and CHO as fuels to resynthesize ATP.

3 Moderately intense exercise requires a mixture of CHO and fat as fuel.

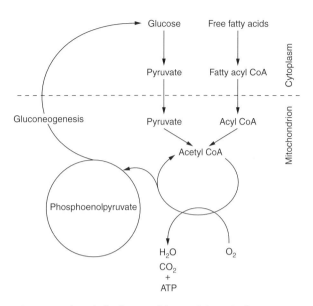

Fig. 5.1 Both carbohydrate and fat participate in the energy transfer process of the citric acid cycle. Alternatively, glucose can be synthesized using phosphoenolpyruvate from this cycle. CoA, coenzyme A.

4 Endogenous CHO depletion, promoting fat to become the dominant fuel, leads to a reduction in endurance exercise capacity.

5 Protein is not a significant exercise fuel under normal physiological conditions.

Energy-rich phosphates

ATP may be sufficient for 2–3 s of sprinting and the CrP pool may resynthesize ATP at a high rate for another 5–10 s at full speed. Athletes have tried to increase the amount of ATP and CrP in muscle by specific training regimes, such as short-distance high-intensity interval sprinting. However, studies have shown that improvements – if any – are only small. Until recently, it was believed that it was not possible to manipulate the energy-rich phosphate pool by nutritional intervention. However, recent research, in which creatine was supplemented to athletes in amounts of 20–30 g for a period of 4–5 days, has shown that power output during highly intense exercise may be significantly increased. The mechanisms suggested to play a role are:

1 increase in total muscle creatine content;

2 higher rate of CrP turnover;

3   reduced ammonia production;
4   faster relaxation of muscle after contraction.

Creatine is a normal component of red meat and is produced in the body. The total body content in a 70 kg person amounts to 120 g. The amount recommended to be ingested by supplements, i.e. 20 g · day^{-1}, may be considered to be supraphysiological. This amount equals that present in a meat portion of 5 kg. A higher rate of CrP turnover means that more CrP is continuously available to supply energy for the resynthesis of ADP to ATP. As a consequence, the ADP concentration will drop less dramatically, resulting in less breakdown of ADP to adenosine monophosphate (AMP) and finally ammonia. Based on the data currently available, it is suggested that creatine supplementation may improve sprint and middle-distance exercise by supporting a high power output, but is inefficient in affecting endurance exercise performance. More research is needed before we can make definite statements about the possible benefits of oral creatine and establish supplementation guidelines for cycling performances of <3 mins. Creatine is not on the International Olympic Committee doping list.

Carbohydrate

In the body, CHO is stored as long chains of glucose units in the liver and the muscles, and is called glycogen. In sedentary people, the glycogen content in the liver approximates 100 g and muscle glycogen may amount to as much as 300 g. Liver glycogen is broken down to supply glucose to the blood in periods of fasting, such as overnight. By this mechanism, blood glucose can be maintained at normal physiological levels. Liver glycogen is restored after consuming a meal. The monosaccharides glucose and fructose, resulting from the digestion of CHO, enter the liver by the portal circulation and are partly taken up to resynthesize glycogen. The rest of the monosaccharides leave the liver in the blood stream and circulate through the body where they are either oxidized or incorporated in the muscle glycogen pool, or converted to fat. During physical exercise, a number of metabolic and hormonal stimuli lead to an increased uptake of blood glucose by the active muscle fibres. At the same time the liver is activated to break down liver glycogen in order to supply glucose to the blood, with the goal of maintaining a normal blood glucose level. Thus, liver glycogen availability is a key factor in avoiding the development of hypoglycaemia during endurance cycling.

Muscle glycogen is broken down rapidly during highly intense exercise such as interval training, tempo training sessions, competitive middle-distance time trials and high-intensity interval-type events such as indoor track cycling competitions. During anaerobic work, the rate of muscle glycogen breakdown to supply glucose for glycolysis may be so high that fast-twitch muscle fibres become depleted within 10–15 min or within 4–6 middle-distance repetitions lasting 1–3 min. The reason is that the ATP requirement is extremely high. Glycolysis proceeds at full speed, resulting in an accumulation of pyruvate before its entrance in the slower-functioning citric acid cycle. As a result, by a mass action process, much of the pyruvate is converted to lactic acid, which is transported out of the muscle and to some degree will be consumed by the slow-twitch muscle fibres within the same muscle. Thus, anaerobic work is highly uneconomical with respect to the amount of glycogen broken down to resynthesize ATP. With aerobic work, where most of the pyruvate enters the citric acid cycle and is oxidized, the rate of glycogen depletion is 18 times lower (1 mol glucose becomes 2 mol ATP in anaerobic metabolism and 36 mol ATP when fully aerobically metabolized)!

These data show that time elapses before glycogen stores within active muscle fibres are emptied. Theoretically, a total muscle glycogen store of 300 g in sedentary people and up to 500 g in trained athletes who consume a CHO-rich diet would last for 60–90 min of exercise. However, the total glycogen pool will never be exclusively available to those muscle groups which are dominantly active during repetitive motor skills, such as the leg muscles in cycling. Therefore, performance capacity may be decreased in highly intense exercise events such as local short-circuit courses after 45–60 min, whereas a limiting role of glycogen in less intense events, such as endurance cycling or triathlon, may first appear after about 70–90 min. The same effects will appear during high-intensity interval bicycle training sessions, compared to moderate-intensity endurance sessions.

In any of the three cases, the effect of CHO depletion will be the same: the muscle relies increasingly on fat as a fuel and as a result, the exercise intensity drops.

Alternatively, exercise intensity can be maintained at a higher level as long as sufficient CHO in the form of glycogen and/or blood glucose remains available. Attempts have been made to increase muscle and liver glycogen levels by a combination of reduced training volume and increased CHO consumption, focusing on starchy-type foods and at the same time reducing fat intake and training volume (Fig. 5.2). The first factor will reduce daily glycogen utilization, while the second increases daily glycogen storage. It has been shown that such a combination significantly augments glycogen storage and, as a result, the cyclist is able to work for longer at a specific exercise intensity. In the 1960s this was realized by a regime of a low-CHO diet and exhausting exercise, followed by a high-CHO diet and almost no exercise. Over the years this method has been optimized towards one in which progressive

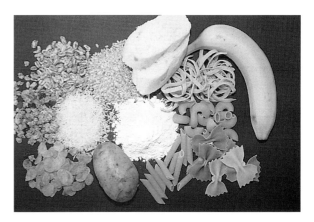

Fig. 5.2 Different types of high-carbohydrate foods.

reduction in training volume (tapering) is combined with a high CHO intake (Fig. 5.3).

An additional measure of optimizing endurance cycling performance is intake of CHO immediately

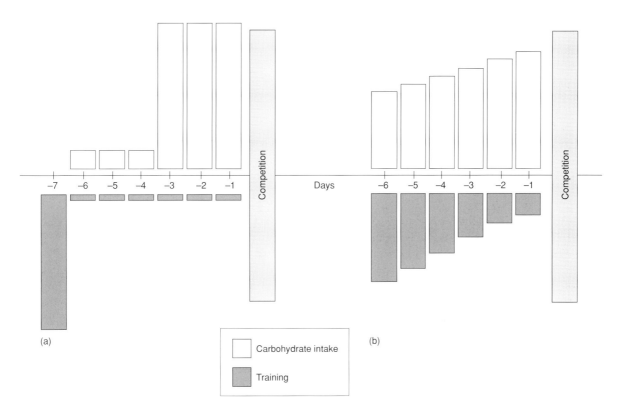

Days

Carbohydrate intake

Training

(a)

(b)

Fig. 5.3 (a) The classic and (b) moderate (tapering) supercompensation protocols as methods of optimizing glycogen storage in the liver and muscle.

before and regularly during exercise. This has been shown to increase blood glucose levels significantly, to augment the respiratory quotient (a sign of enhanced CHO utilization for energy production) and to spare endogenous CHO pools. The latter finding results from studies in which carbon-13 (C^{13})-labelled CHO was ingested during exercise. The appearance of the C^{13} label in the carbon dioxide of expired air can be measured and serves as a tool to calculate oxidation of orally ingested CHO. Based on the measurements of the respiratory quotient it is possible to calculate total CHO oxidation. In this way it has been shown that the total amount of oxidized CHO does not increase during highly intense exercise after CHO ingestion, while oral CHO is oxidized. The conclusion is that endogenous CHO oxidation is reduced when oral CHO is oxidized. In other words, endogenous CHO pools are less utilized when oral CHO is supplied during exercise. From these studies we have learned that the maximal rate at which oral CHO is oxidized amounts to $0.6–1.2 \text{ g} \cdot \text{min}^{-1}$. This amount also gives an indication of the optimal amount which should be ingested during intense endurance cycling: $40–70 \text{ g} \cdot \text{h}^{-1}$.

Additionally, it has been observed that different types of soluble CHO are oxidized equally effectively. An exception may be fructose, which is oxidized at a lower rate and may induce gastrointestinal upset when ingested in quantities of $>30 \text{ g} \cdot \text{l}^{-1}$. Some concern has been raised from studies which showed that hypoglycaemia may develop by a rebound mechanism when CHO is ingested 45 min before exercise in resting conditions. Such a procedure rapidly increases blood glucose – and insulin. When exercise is started, the elevated insulin blocks glycogen degradation in the liver and the liberation of fatty acids from adipose tissue. At the same time muscle glucose uptake increases and uptake of fatty acids diminishes, due to the reduced supply from the fat cells to the blood plasma. As a result, blood glucose may fall rapidly to hypoglycaemic levels. However, the results of these studies should be interpreted with care. Athletes normally do not compete after an overnight fast and should perform warming-up exercises before the start of the race. In a study where different types of CHO were ingested immediately before an endurance event, during warming up, we could not find any negative effect on blood glucose. Meanwhile, a number of studies have shown that well-timed pre-exercise CHO intake may improve performance, probably by optimizing liver and muscle glycogen levels.

In summary:

1 Highly intense exercise rapidly depletes muscle glycogen.

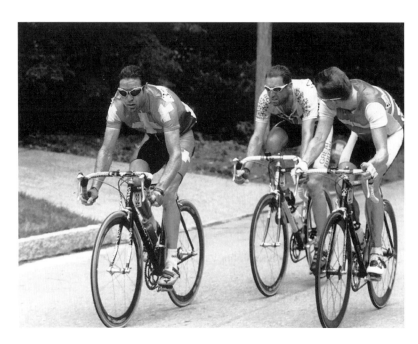

Fig. 5.4 Atlanta 1996: road race. Richard Pascal (SUI), first; Sciandri Mazimilian (GBR), second; and Sorensen Rolf (DEN), third. © Allsport / Mike Powell.

2 Low muscle glycogen levels coincide with a reduction in performance capacity.

3 Sufficient liver glycogen is the key factor for maintaining normal blood glucose levels.

4 Both liver and muscle glycogen resynthesis depend on the supply of glucose units, mainly from food.

5 CHO-rich meals augment body CHO stores and delay fatigue.

6 CHO ingestion immediately before and during exercise spares endogenous CHO and delays fatigue.

7 Fructose is utilized slowly during exercise compared to glucose, sucrose, maltose and maltodextrins.

Fat

The importance of fat as a substrate during athletic performance depends on the degree of exercise stress as well as on the availability of CHO. In non-trained subjects body fat content may be 20–35% for females and 10–20% for males. Fat is stored in the body as triglycerides in fat cells and in small fat droplets within the muscle fibres. Trained athletes have less body fat: 5–15% in males and 10–25% in females. During physical exercise free fatty acids (FFA) and glycerol are mobilized from the adipocytes in adipose tissue. Both enter the blood stream. At low to moderate blood FFA levels, the uptake of FFA in muscle is influenced by the blood plasma concentration. However, this effect is only present at a low plasma FFA concentration. At higher blood FFA levels there is no further increase, probably because of limitations in muscle FFA uptake across the muscle cell membrane. Thus, FFA uptake by muscle may reach its maximum after 20–40 min of endurance exercise, when blood fatty acids have increased to a level of $0.6–1.0 \text{ mmol} \cdot \text{l}^{-1}$. In this situation the extraction of FFA from plasma by muscle is only 15–20% of the total supply.

It has long been thought that augmenting plasma fatty acids further, by supplying lipolysis-stimulating agents such as caffeine and theophylline or by oral ingestion of fat, may further enhance muscle FFA uptake and oxidation.

However, scientific data point to the fact that endurance-trained muscle cannot be stimulated to increase fat utilization by such measures. In contrast, CHO uptake and oxidation increase with greater exercise intensity, when FFA oxidation has reached a plateau. In this respect it is interesting to note a care-

ful study in highly trained cyclists who were depleted in one situation and glycogen-repleted by maltodextrin ingestion in another. When glycogen-depleted, blood glucose fell to hypoglycaemic levels and lactate was low as a result of poor CHO availability. At the same time, fat metabolism was maximally activated, leading to dramatically increased blood fatty acid, glycerol and ketone levels. However, performance dropped to <50% of maximal capacity in this condition. With adequate glycogen levels and regular CHO intake during exercise, cyclists could maintain a work output of 70% maximal achieved work load (W_{max}) equivalent to ±80% $V_{O_{2max}}$, for 2 h without problems. This indicates that, for optimal performance, sufficient CHO and fat should be available as fuel.

Apart from FFA derived from fat cells in adipose tissue, muscle may also contribute significantly to FFA supply during exercise. Most probably, the increased fat oxidation observed in periods of CHO shortage during intensive endurance exercise, comes from the triglycerides stored intramuscularly. Since long-chain fatty acid uptake in the mitochondria is mediated by carnitine, it has also been suggested that L-carnitine supplementation increases fat utilization, However, carefully performed studies could not demonstrate such an effect. Therefore, it is concluded that oral L-carnitine supplements have no enhancing effect on fat transport and oxidation in healthy trained individuals. Since fat uptake by muscle is limited, it makes no sense to supply oral fat during exercise. In fact, a large body of evidence has shown that CHO, not fat, is the limiting nutrient for intense endurance exercise. Since fat reduces the gastric emptying rate, initiates small intestinal contractions and is involved in gastrointestinal problems during exercise, it is recommended that one should consume low-fat foods before and during intense exercise. This recommendation is not valid for less intense sport events where CHO availability is not limiting, such as cycle touring or orienteering.

Protein

The human body has no metabolically available protein stores, unlike fat and carbohydrate. Apart from a small amount of circulating and intracellular free amino acids (AA), all proteins in the body are functional proteins. This means that they are part of cell or

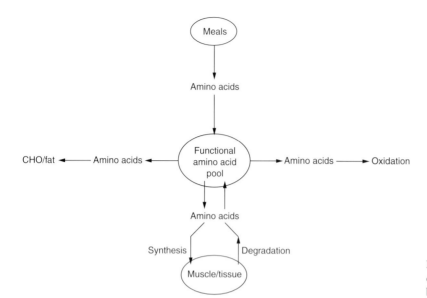

Fig. 5.5 The fate of amino acids derived from food or from the breakdown of tissue within the body.

tissue structures or act as metabolic regulators such as enzymes or hormones. Any AA from the diet which are not incorporated in new functional proteins or are used to maintain existing protein structures are doomed to be either oxidized or converted to fat. AA which result from the digestion of consumed protein or from the breakdown of functional proteins in the body will enter the free AA pool in plasma and cells. From this pool AA will be used for energy or synthesis processes (Fig. 5.5).

The composition of the AA pool is kept within a narrow range. Any shortage of non-essential AA will stimulate the production of these AA. A shortage of essential AA, on the other hand, cannot be compensated for by synthesis through the body, since the body cannot synthesize essential AA.

There are only two ways of compensating for a shortage in essential AA:
1 to increase protein consumption, especially of proteins which have a high content of essential AA, such as high-biological-value proteins like milk, protein from egg, meat and fish and their combinations with vegetable plant proteins;
2 to break down body proteins containing these AA.

This second point has been suggested as one of the reasons for increased muscle breakdown in periods of inadequate AA supply. Exercise is known to be associated with changes in the AA pool, primarily because of oxidation of AA which increases with

increasing exercise intensity, especially in a situation of glycogen depletion. The AA which are oxidized are mostly the branched-chain AA (BCAA) leucine, isoleucine and valine. As a result of the oxidation, the nitrogen group is liberated and converted to ammonia ($NH^2 + H^+ \rightarrow NH_3$), a substance known to be involved in reducing the rate of a number of metabolic steps in energy metabolism and also suggested to be involved in the development of fatigue. Many studies have shown that the best way of preventing considerable AA oxidation is to take measures to ensure sufficient CHO availability.

Recently, BCAA have attracted special interest. The fact that these AA are preferably oxidized by muscle was interpreted by some scientists as demonstrating that they are a welcome energy source for exercising individuals. In other words, BCAA were promoted for consumption during exercise. However, the scientists overlooked the fact that increased BCAA oxidation leads to increased ammonia production, which is an undesirable metabolic event during exercise. Additionally, they did not take into account the fact that CHO supplementation has a much more powerful effect on both performance and protein utilization, since CHO oxidation frees more energy for muscle contraction.

An additional argument to promote BCAA supplementation is that they reduce central fatigue. Although this may sound contradictory, knowing the effects of ammonia production and possible fatigue, the hypothesis underlying this assumption is as follows: as a result of oxidation during exercise, the concentration of BCAA in blood plasma decreases. The concentration of other AA in relation to BCAA increases, for example, tryptophan, which is a precursor for the formation of serotonin in the brain. Serotonin induces relaxation, sleep and feelings of tiredness. Since the transport mechanism for BCAA and tryptophan at the blood–brain barrier is the same, more tryptophan is taken up by the brain and more serotonin may be formed. Supplementation of BCAA, maintaining normal BCAA levels, is suggested to prevent this increased tryptophan uptake. However, despite a first positive report of BCAA supplementation in slow marathon runners, no single well-controlled study has proved that consuming BCAA during endurance exercise is of any benefit. In contrast, there are more reasons to expect that BCAA supplementation during exercise may be a disadvantage to the athlete.

Other AA, such as arginine, ornithine and tyrosine, have been postulated to affect hormone levels and therefore performance. It should be noted that the possible hormone effects were mostly observed in animal studies and only with extremely high AA dosages. Further, effects in humans, if any, are all within the range of the normal hormone fluctuations caused by daily biorhythms and food intake. Therefore, any single AA supplementation in periods of intense exercise, with the goal of promoting the production of anabolic hormones or catecholamines, seems to be ineffective. Nevertheless, those athletes who have a strong belief in these substances may experience a positive placebo effect – at the cost of a considerable financial investment.

Because of increased AA oxidation in periods of intensive training, athletes have a higher daily protein requirement (g · kg^{-1} body weight · day^{-1}) compared to sedentary people who require about 1 g · kg^{-1} body weight · day^{-1}. The question remains whether this increased requirement justifies the need for protein supplementation. The answer is that this is not the case in endurance athletes who have high energy intakes. For example, in studies performed during the Tour de France, it was observed that mean daily energy intake amounted to ±27.3 MJ · day^{-1} (±6500 kcal · day^{-1}). Some 12% of this energy intake resulted from protein intake, as much as 3 g · kg^{-1} body weight ·

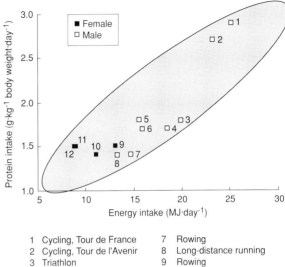

1 Cycling, Tour de France
2 Cycling, Tour de l'Avenir
3 Triathlon
4 Cycling, amateur
5 Speedskating, marathon
6 Swimming
7 Rowing
8 Long-distance running
9 Rowing
10 Cycling, amateur
11 Long-distance running
12 Swimming

Fig. 5.6 There is a close relation between the consumption of protein and other essential nutrients and total daily energy intake. This graph represents the data from a large number of Olympic athletes and participants in world and European championships. Reproduced with permission.

day^{-1}. Nitrogen balance studies have shown that, in cyclists who become glycogen-depleted on a daily basis, the protein requirement may be as high as 1.8 g · kg^{-1} body weight · day^{-1}. Based on many other studies, it is suggested that the protein requirement of endurance athletes may range from 1.2 to 1.8 g · kg^{-1} body weight · day^{-1} (Fig. 5.6). Thus, in general, cyclists who increase their food intake to compensate for increased energy utilization will be in positive nitrogen balance. The exceptions are those situations where low food intake, either through dieting or illness, takes place. In this case, the athlete should be advised to enhance protein intake using high-protein foods or supplements.

Fluid and electrolytes

The body of an average 75 kg athlete contains about 60% or 45 l water. Muscle comprises approximately 70–75% water, whereas fat contains only about 10–15%. From this it may be concluded that lean endurance athletes have a relatively high water content. The normal route of fluid ingested orally is, firstly, appearance in the blood, than transfer into the interstitial fluid and, lastly, into the intracellular fluid. The route of continuing fluid loss by urine, diarrhoea or sweat is exactly the opposite. Fluid loss from the body comes initially from the blood plasma. This results in additional flux from the interstitial fluid to compensate for the reduction in plasma volume. Lastly, with ongoing losses, the interstitial fluid is maintained at a certain level by water flux out of the intracellular compartment. Thus, during early periods of dehydration it is primarily the plasma volume which is mostly affected, whereas during long-lasting dehydration, it is increasingly the intracellular fluid.

Dehydration of the body leads to a number of physiological changes which impair thermoregulation and performance capacity, especially during exercise in the heat. Therefore, it is of great concern that fluid loss in exercising athletes is minimized. Because glycogen-bound water is liberated when glycogen is broken down to supply glucose for energy metabolism and because substrates are oxidized, leading to the production of metabolic water, some weight loss may occur during endurance exercise without there being any consequences for the hydration status of the body. Any weight loss exceeding ±1 kg body weight may reflect net water loss from the body. Such a change in body weight is the best measure for athletes of whether fluid intake during exercise is sufficient or not.

With sweating, electrolytes are excreted. Studies have shown that the amount excreted depends on the blood mineral level, training status and sweat rate. The average content of electrolytes in muscle cell water, blood plasma and sweat is given in Table 5.2.

From this table it can be concluded that sweat contains considerably fewer electrolytes than plasma, with the exception of potassium and magnesium. As a result, blood mineral levels increase when sweat loss is great and no fluid is ingested to compensate for the losses. When large amounts of water are consumed to compensate for sweat loss, blood plasma is diluted. Blood osmolality and electrolyte levels may fall in this condition. This situation may be pronounced during ultra-endurance events (>3–4 h) where large amounts of water are drunk. For this reason, many commercially available sports drinks contain electrolytes at levels comparable to sweat electrolyte content. There is no evidence that inclusion of electrolytes in drinks improve performance, but there is good evidence that

Table 5.2 Average concentrations ($mg \cdot l^{-1}$) of major electrolytes in sweat compared to intra- and extracellular water.

	Sweat	Intracellular	Plasma
Sodium	413–1091	230	2990–3565
Potassium	121–225	5850	125–215
Calcium	13–67	very low	42–58
Magnesium	4–34	182	8–18
Chloride	533–1495	284	3408–3905

the addition of sodium to sport rehydration drinks, together with moderate amounts of CHO ($30–80 \text{ g} \cdot l^{-1}$) improves water absorption and retention. Additionally, the CHO supports glucose availability.

Consumption of drinks during exercise with electrolytes at levels considerably higher than are lost with sweat is not recommended. This may increase blood osmolality, which will reduce sweat rate and thus affect thermoregulation negatively. Additionally, the kidneys will be put under stress to excrete electrolytes in a situation where urine flow is extremely low.

In general, it is recommended that fluid replacement drinks for athletes contain $30–80 \text{ g CHO} \cdot l^{-1}$, and not more than 1100 mg sodium, 1500 mg chloride, 225 mg potassium, 100 mg magnesium and 225 mg Ca^{2+}. The drink should not be strongly hypertonic compared to blood plasma: it should have an osmolality of $<500 \text{ mosmol} \cdot l^{-1}$, preferably ≤ 300 $mosmol \cdot l^{-1}$. Many sports drinks fall within these ranges and have been proven to result in high gastric emptying and faster intestinal absorption rate than tap and mineral water (Fig. 5.7).

Guidelines for practice

Based on the information given above and the recommendations which resulted from a recent symposium on aspects of nutrition for endurance athletes, the following guidelines can be given.*

* These recommendations are reproduced with permission of the Isostar Sport Nutrition Foundation, Papendal Symposium 1997, *Insider* Vol 5, Part 1: *Nutrition for Endurance Sport; from Theory to Practice* by A. Jeukendrup and F. Brouns.

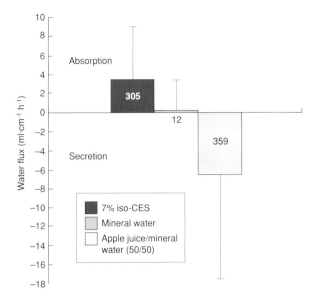

Fig. 5.7 Absorption of a 7% carbohydrate–electrolyte solution (CES), mineral water and a combination of mineral water and apple juice. The CES was absorbed significantly faster than the mineral water. The fruit juice–mineral water combination resulted in a temporary net secretion, probably caused by a secretion-inducing substance from the apple.

Pre-competition nutritional guidelines

1 CHO load using a moderate (tapering) supercompensation diet.

2 Ensure a CHO intake of about 600 g · day^{-1} during the 3 days before the race. Intake of more than this amount may not increase glycogen storage and is therefore not necessary.

3 Drink plenty of fluids on the days before the race, to ensure that you are well hydrated at the start of the event. If substantial sweat losses are expected during the race (see the discussion on sports drinks, above), add a small amount of sodium chloride (about the tip of a teaspoon of table salt per litre) to your drink or use a sports drink containing 500–1000 mg sodium · l^{-1}.

4 Avoid foods with a high dietary fibre content on the days before the competition to prevent gastrointestinal problems.

5 Eat a CHO-rich pre-event meal 2–4 h before a race to ensure adequate levels of glycogen in the liver. Before short races ingest easily digestible CHO foods or energy drinks. Before long races eat semisolid or solid food such as energy bars or bread, and keep the intake of fat and protein low.

6 Some individuals may develop rebound hypoglycaemia following a high-CHO meal or drink before a race. These individuals should delay eating CHO until during the warm-up, or until the last 3–5 min before the start of the race.

Guidelines for nutrition during exercise

1 During intense exercise lasting >45 min a CHO drink should be ingested. This may improve performance by reducing or delaying fatigue.

2 Consume 40–60 g of CHO for each hour of exercise. This can be optimally combined with fluid in quantities related to need, which is determined by environmental conditions, individual sweat rates and gastrointestinal tolerance.

3 During exercise of <45 min duration it is not necessary to consume CHO.

4 The type of soluble CHO (glucose, sucrose, glucose polymer, etc.) ingested does not appear to make much difference when ingested in low to moderate quantities; fructose and galactose are less effective. Insoluble CHO sources are relatively slowly absorbed and oxidized, and are therefore not recommended for high-intensity events.

5 Cyclists should drink beverages containing CHO, rather than water, during the whole event.

6 Avoid drinks which have extremely high CHO contents (>20%) and those with a high osmolality (>500 mosmol · kg^{-1}) because fluid delivery will be hampered and gastrointestinal problems may occur.

7 Try to predict the fluid loss during endurance events of >90 min. The volume of fluid to be ingested should in principle at least equal the predicted fluid loss. While exercising in warm weather with low humidity, athletes need to drink more to replace sweat loss and the drinks can be dilute. In cold weather, athletes require less fluid volume to maintain fluid balance but will still require the CHO to maintain blood glucose levels, therefore the CHO content of the drinks can be more concentrated.

8 Large volumes of a drink stimulate gastric emptying more than small volumes. Therefore, we recommend that athletes ingest a fluid volume of 6–8 ml · kg^{-1} body weight, 3–5 min before the start to prime the stomach, followed by smaller amounts (2–3 ml · kg^{-1} body weight) every 15–20 min.

9 The volume of fluid athletes can ingest is usually limited. Cyclists should practise drinking while exercising as the volume the gastrointestinal tract will tolerate can be increased by training.

10 After a period of frequent drinking, the stomach may feel empty and uncomfortable. If this occurs, it may be wise to eat easily digested solid food. During long, low-intensity competitions solid food can be eaten in the early stages of the event.

11 Factors such as high fibre and high protein content and high CHO concentration and osmolality have been associated with the development of gastrointestinal symptoms during exercise, and thus should be avoided.

Postexercise nutritional guidelines

1 To maximize glycogen resynthesis, it is recommended that in the first 2 h after exercise 100 g of CHO is ingested in the form of liquids or easily digestible solid or semisolid food. Thereafter $25 \, g \cdot h^{-1}$ is recommended. In all, about $10 \, g \, CHO \cdot kg^{-1}$ body weight should be eaten within 24 h.

2 CHO sources with a moderate-to-high glycaemic index should be eaten if the next performance has to take place within 24 h.

3 Adding a protein powder to the CHO consumed during the first hours postexercise may stimulate glycogen recovery rates.

4 There is no proven benefit in consuming single amino acid supplements or mixtures of amino acids.

5 Adding >500 mg sodium to postexercise rehydration beverages improves fluid retention and fluid balance recovery.

Minerals

Apart from minerals lost with sweat, loss occurs daily with urine and a non-absorbed fraction is lost in the stool. Daily mineral requirements should be met by eating a variety of foods, of which vegetables, milk products and meat are especially good mineral suppliers. Cyclists who consume daily large amounts of food normally have a good mineral intake. As with protein (see Fig. 5.6), there is a close relationship between energy intake and mineral supply. More food supplies more minerals.

The exceptions are those situations where athletes cannot eat enough food due to poor availability, lack of appetite or when dieting to lose weight. In these situations it is advisable to supplement with a low-dose preparation containing iron, magnesium, Ca^{2+} and zinc in amounts not exceeding the recommended daily allowance (Table 5.3).

Mineral status is difficult to determine. Since most minerals are bound to, or part of, functional systems and structures, the amount immediately available for metabolism is in fact small. Most of the metabolic mineral pool is present in blood and interstitial fluid.

Table 5.3 Recommended dietary allowances for minerals (mg). NRC, National Research Council USA; DGE, Deutsche Gesellschaft für Ernährung-Germany.

   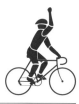

Age (years)	Magnesium	Calcium	Phosphorus	Iron	Zinc
Males					
15–18/15–18	400/400	1200/1200	1200/1600	12/12	15/15
19–24/19–25	350/350	1200/1000	1200/1500	10/10	15/15
25–50/25–51	350/350	800/900	800/1400	10/10	10/15
Females					
15–18/15–18	300/350	1200/1200	1200/1600	15/15	12/12
19–24/19–25	280/300	1000/1000	1200/1500	15/15	12/12
25–50/25–51	280/300	800/900	800/1400	15/15	12/12
NRC/DGE	NRC/DGE	NRC/DGE	NRC/DGE	NRC/DGE	NRC/DGE

Magnesium

Magnesium (Mg^{2+}) is an essential mineral for about 300 enzymes and plays an important role in neuro-muscular transmission. Almost all metabolically available Mg^{2+} is located in the extracellular pool. Any change in this pool is caused by either supply from food and drinks or by losses in urine and sweat. Sweat losses are generally small but may become significant with prolonged sweating. Low resting as well as exercise Mg^{2+} levels have repeatedly been reported in endurance athletes. Marginal Mg^{2+} status has been suggested to be associated with impaired energy metabolism, decreased performance and with the occurrence of muscle cramps, although this has never been confirmed in the case of exercise-induced cramp. Low plasma Mg^{2+} levels may be the result of exercise-induced Mg^{2+} shifts into red blood cells and fat tissue. Therefore it is difficult to conclude that a low plasma Mg^{2+} is representative of a poor Mg^{2+} status.

The Mg^{2+} content of food varies widely. Vegetables, exotic fruits, bananas, nuts, mushrooms and grains are relatively rich in Mg^{2+}, while fish, meat and milk are relatively poor. Data concerning Mg^{2+} intake in athletes are scarce. A recent study, however, indicated a close relationship between Mg^{2+} intake and energy intake. Endurance athletes in particular were observed to have daily Mg^{2+} intakes which were significantly above the daily recommended allowance for sedentary people.

Calcium

The human body contains about 1200 g calcium (Ca^{2+}), of which approximately 99% is within the skeleton. Only a fraction (1%) is present in extra-cellular fluid and intracellular structures of the soft tissues. This small fraction represents the metabolically available pool. Plasma Ca^{2+} is maintained in a narrow range, mainly by hormones which control absorption, secretion and bone metabolism. When Ca^{2+} intake is too low, plasma Ca^{2+} levels remain constant, at the cost of reduced absorption into the bone and normal or increased release from the bone. Therefore, the plasma Ca^{2+} level does not indicate the true Ca^{2+} status of the body. Scientific studies have shown that female athletes may suffer from stress fractures and/or reduced bone density. This athletic osteoporosis has been suggested to be caused by exercise stress-induced depression of the oestrogen status, especially in female long-distance runners. However, in female cyclists these observations have not been made, probably because cyclists have higher energy intake as well as greater body weight. Also, Ca^{2+} intake varies with the quantity and composition of the diet. Dairy products form the major source of Ca^{2+} intake. Nuts, pulses, some green vegetables (broccoli) and seafood, as well as Ca^{2+} from water, may further contribute.

Phosphorus

Phosphorus is the counterpart of Ca^{2+} in bone formation. Virtually all phosphorus circulating in blood and present in tissues exists in the metabolically active form as the phosphate (PO_4^{3-}) molecule. About 85% of the total body store is present in the skeleton. The remainder is distributed between extracellular and intracellular space in soft tissue. Phosphorus intake, and consequently tissue supply via the blood, is known to affect bone formation. Therefore, intake of both minerals is advised to be in balance. Phosphorus is an important cofactor for a large number of enzymes. Since exercise results in sweat loss and haemoconcentration, it may enhance plasma phosphate levels. Phosphate losses through sweat itself, however, are negligible. Phosphorus is especially present in protein-rich foods such as milk, meat, poultry and fish, as well as in cereal products. Increases in daily energy intake will normally also increase phosphorus intake. Therefore, phosphorus deficiencies have not been observed in cyclists.

Iron

Iron is an important constituent of haemoglobin, myoglobin and a number of enzymes. As such, the availability of iron is important for oxygen binding and transport as well as for energy transfer. About 30% of total iron is found in storage forms as ferritin and haemosiderin and a small part as transferrin. Therefore these iron stores can serve as indicators of iron status. Poor iron status is indicated by low levels of serum ferritin, increased red cell protoporphyrin levels, reduced transferrin saturation levels and reduced haemoglobin levels. With inadequate iron intake, the storage form will be the first to be affected. With prolonged iron shortage, haemoglobin production will finally be affected, resulting in iron-deficiency anaemia, which will reduce oxygen transport capacity and thus may affect endurance performance capacity.

A substantial number of studies have shown decreased iron stores in endurance athletes. This was indicated by reduced bone marrow iron, low serum/plasma ferritin levels and enhanced iron-binding capacity. Some data may be misleading, since stressful exercise has been shown to result in temporarily increased serum ferritin levels. Thus, serum ferritin levels obtained shortly after intense endurance exercise may no longer accurately reflect body iron stores. Significant amounts of iron may be lost with sweat. This may explain the effects of frequent endurance training sessions on haemoglobin levels. The effect of exercise on iron absorption in the gut, especially ultra-endurance activities which reduce intestinal blood flow and may affect other transport processes, remains largely unknown. Also unknown is the magnitude to which decreased iron stores in athletes increase iron absorption, as has been observed in sedentary individuals.

Recent studies have shown that endurance exercise may lead to gastrointestinal bleeding. As a result, increased faecal haemoglobin and iron losses have been observed. However, this was mainly the case in endurance runners and significantly less so in cyclists. Red meat, liver, poultry, dark green vegetables and cereals (especially iron-fortified products) are the main sources of iron intake. Haem iron in meat is the best absorbable iron source. Iron absorption from non-haem sources is less and can be further decreased by other food/meal constituents. Vitamin C enhances inorganic iron absorption, while dietary fibre, tea, coffee and Ca^{2+} phosphate reduce absorption. The recommended/safe daily intake for iron is shown in Table 5.3. It is assumed that the required daily intake for athletes exceeds this recommended daily allowance. Research should be done to establish the true requirements of athletes.

Zinc

Zinc is present in relatively large amounts in bone and muscle. However, these stores are not metabolically

available. The body pool of readily available zinc, mainly in blood, is small and has a rapid turnover. Zinc is involved in the growth and development of tissues, especially muscle, as it is an essential substance in numerous enzymes involved in major metabolic pathways. Recent studies have indicated that zinc may also play a crucial role in resistance against infections and illness. Since plasma zinc represents to a large extent the readily available zinc pool, it can be understood that any rapid change in plasma volume, due to the performance of physical exercise, will affect plasma zinc status. This can occur either by a plasma volume decrease, due to fluid shifts into muscle or to dehydration (which will increase the plasma zinc concentration), or by a plasma volume

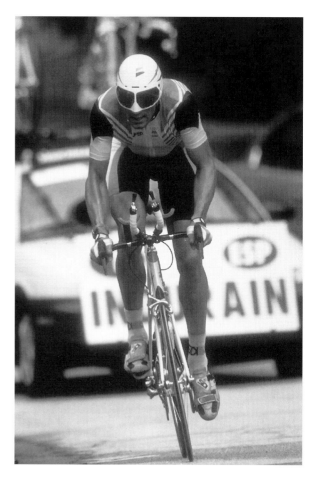

Fig. 5.8 Atlanta 1996: individual time trial. Miguel Indurain (ESP), first. © Allsport / Bruno Bade.

increase in the postexercise phase, caused by water and sodium retention (which will decrease zinc concentration). Apart from these effects it may be assumed that functional zinc shifts between tissues may occur due to exercise.

For these reasons it is difficult to determine the effect of exercise on zinc status as indicated by plasma zinc levels. (Plasma zinc was observed to increase significantly over several weeks of cycling in the Tour de France. However, it is not known what the implication of this observation is.) Nevertheless, exercise may increase zinc requirements because of increased losses with urine and sweat as a result of the exercise stress. Meat, liver and seafood are major zinc sources in the diet. Additional zinc may be derived from milk, cereals and muesli. High-CHO foods, especially refined sources, are poor zinc sources. Zinc intake in athletes is observed to be closely related to total energy intake. The recommended safe daily intake for zinc is given in Table 5.3.

Mineral replacement and supplementation

From the previous paragraphs it can be concluded that mineral intake in endurance cyclists will be sufficient in most cases and that supplementation for cyclists who eat a well-balanced diet, containing sufficient amounts of meat, fruits, vegetables, cereals and whole-grain products, will not be a priority.

In this respect it is still an open question whether the recommended daily allowance established for sedentary people is also adequate for athletes who, due to exercise, may lose substantial amounts of minerals with urine and sweat. Mineral replacement by adding minerals to rehydration drinks is acceptable and safe as long as the mineral levels do not exceed the upper levels reported for whole-body sweat (see Table 5.2). Although substantial amounts of iron can be lost with sweat, there is to our knowledge no rationale to replace this mineral in drinks which are to be consumed during exercise.

Chapter 6

Medical problems in

road cycling

Overuse injuries

Overuse injuries are chronic, uncontrolled, overload, microtraumatic events. Overuse injuries occur over a period of time, when forces applied to a structure are increased faster than the structure can adapt, or exceed its limits of adaptation. Too many miles, or too intense miles (especially hills and big gears), often cause overuse injury in cyclists. Less commonly, excessive spinning may cause problems.

Overuse injuries also occur when the bicycle is not correctly adjusted. Riders with anatomical variants may require non-standard configurations of their equipment, for example in the case of leg-length discrepancy the use of asymmetrically positioned cleats may be advisable.

Overuse injuries can be graded according to pain persistence:

Grade 1: pain only after activity;
Grade 2: pain starts during activity;
Grade 3: pain persists the next day;
Grade 4: constant pain.

Some body types or anatomy predispose to certain overuse injuries. For example:

1 Leg-length discrepancy is not usually associated with problems in the general or recreational rider population unless the difference between the legs exceeds 6 mm. However, long-distance riders or racers may experience leg-length discrepancy-related problems with as little as 3 mm difference.
2 A wide pelvis places the knees farther apart and stresses the lateral (outside) structures of the knee.
3 Excessive foot pronation is associated with medial (inside) knee pain.
4 The shin bone, or tibia, is twisted internally as a normal human variant in many people. This twist results in a tendency of the feet to turn inward. Trying to ride with toes pointed straight ahead may cause discomfort of the medial knee.
5 Unbalanced muscles or other anatomical variants may lead to abnormal tracking of the kneecap.

Treatment principles

In the first instance, overuse injuries should be prevented by applying general principles which are common to all sports. Allow the body sufficient time to adapt. Increase activity levels gradually and allow periods of rest and adaptation, for example, by alternating heavy and light workouts. A warm-up and cool-down and stretching before and after may help. In bicycling, warm-up, cool-down and stretching are more important for track racers than for road riders.

The following treatment methods, as well as stretching and strengthening programmes, are discussed under treatment options later in this chapter.

1 Adjust activity to allow healing. Adjusted activity may be preferable to complete rest.
2 Reduce inflammation. Ice, oral non-steroidal anti-inflammatory drugs (NSAIDs), cortisone injections and physical therapy, including ultrasound, electrical stimulation and contrast baths, are common ways to reduce inflammation.
3 Correct biomechanical stress or external factors. In bicycling, check and modify bicycle fit and cleat placement as necessary. Bicycle fit must be individualized to the injured rider – it may not be the correct position for the average uninjured rider. As an example, consider overuse knee injuries, which are the most common overuse injuries for which cyclists consult a doctor. Basic position considerations are seat and foot position. The seat may be too low or too high, too far forward or too far back. The feet may be too far apart or too close together; too toed in or out; too far forward or too far back in relation to the pedal axle. When the problem is the distance between the feet, correction may be made by:

    (a) changing the cleat position;
    (b) using a different-length bottom bracket axle;
    (c) using cranks with a different offset;
    (d) using a shim between the pedal axle and the crank.

Foot rotation may be a factor. Pedal flotation allows the foot to rotate on the bicycle pedal. This freedom of motion has helped many riders for whom the fixed-cleat position has contributed to knee strain. Too much float may also be harmful: limiting flotation may allow some overuse injuries to improve.

Off-the-bike activities

Other athletic activities may contribute to the cause of overuse injuries or hinder recovery. Running can be especially stressful on the knee. Running up and especially down hills places tremendous pressure on the knee. Running on inclines, such as along the beach or the side of a canted road, places stresses on the medial and lateral knee. Offending activities may need to be curtailed.

Weight training has many benefits; it is also taxing on the body. Many exercises that specifically strengthen the quadriceps – perhaps the most important cycling muscle – also place large loads on the knee-cap where it glides over the thigh bone. Full squats, leg extensions and lunges are particularly gruelling for knee structures. Some weight training may need to be curtailed.

General anatomical classification

Overuse injuries commonly affect four body structures: tendons, bursae, nerves and bones.

1 Tendinitis. Tendons are fibrous cords of tissue which join muscles to bone and allow the muscles to move bones relative to each other at joints. Tendinitis is inflammation or irritation of a tendon. Irritations to the tendon can be caused by different reasons. A fall may bruise a tendon; overuse may strain a tendon; sudden forces or extra-hard efforts may do the same. Pain comes from nerve irritation within the tendon and is a warning sign that something is wrong – the tendon itself may be stretched and swollen, or small parts of it may be torn. Many of the overuse injuries described below, especially those of the knee, are overuse tendon injuries.

2 Bursitis. Bursae are cystic structures that form between surfaces that move over each other, probably to lubricate movement. Sometimes the surface is a tendon, sometimes a bone. Bursitis is inflammation or irritation of a bursa. When one of the surfaces is a tendon, it is often impossible to distinguish between tendinitis and bursitis. The difference between

tendinitis and bursitis in such a situation may be of little relevance, since the treatment of either condition is often the same.

3 Compression neuropathy. A neuropathy is an abnormality of nerve function. Compression pressure on a nerve, or on the blood vessels that supply a nerve, is associated with a number of well-known neuropathies. Common cycling neuropathies includes cyclist's palsy, a neuropathy of the ulnar nerve in the hand, and penile numbness, a common neuropathy related to abnormal function of the pudendal nerve.

4 Stress fracture. A stress fracture is an overuse injury of bone. Beginning with microfractures, untreated stress fractures may proceed to completed or through-and-through fractures. Stress fractures are relatively uncommon in cycling.

Specific injuries

The rest of this section will review specific cycling overuse injuries from the neck down. Considerable attention will be devoted to the knee since firstly, the knee is the most common site for overuse injury in cyclists, and secondly, the bicycle position adjustment for knee injury may be completely different depending on the type of knee injury.

Neck pain

We are concerned here with musculoskeletal pain in the back of the neck. Sometimes neck pain travels upward, causing a headache. Consider a neurological origin and consultation whenever neck pain is associated with upper-extremity symptoms: pain, loss of sensation or loss of power in the arms. Consider urgent or emergency medical consultation when pain in the front of the neck or in the jaw is associated with exercise, as this may be a symptom of cardiac origin.

Causes

Neck pain can follow strain or overuse. The pain may travel to the back of the head and become more generalized. If nerves are involved, it may travel to the arms. It is usually due to:

1 muscle strain and/or spasm;

2 arthritis – usually degenerative (wear-and-tear) osteoarthritis. Strain on the vertebral joints from misalignment, often secondary to disc degeneration, also causes pain;

3 a bulge or herniation of an intervertebral disc. This may cause pain travelling to the arms.

In younger cyclists neck pain is usually due to muscle strain. In older cyclists a combination of muscle strain and degenerative changes is often responsible. Degenerative changes are usually age- and not cycling-related.

Cycling-related neck strain is often associated with long rides. The position on the bike can be important. Cyclists who lack flexibility may find the aerodynamic bent-over racing position uncomfortable. Anything that forces the rider to increase stretch in the neck may cause neck pain.

Women tend to ride bikes with top tubes that are too long. (Most bikes are designed for men; women have relatively longer legs and shorter reaches.)

Jarring from rough mountain-bike riding can be a factor. Road riders who keep their necks and shoulders locked, and who forget to look around, are prone to neck pain.

Neck pain may be non-cycling-related, arising from muscle tension due to stress, anxiety, depression or fatigue, or from poor posture.

Treatment

On-the-bicycle. If neck pain is due to long rides:
1 Allow for a gradual increase in endurance riding. Increase the length of endurance rides no more than 10% per week.
2 Consciously relax the upper body – back, elbows and neck – every few minutes. Change hand position, which will change the neck position and reduce strain.
3 Stretch the neck on the bike. Look around: do not focus only on the pavement directly in front.
4 A helmet is a must for safety, but make sure it is light-weight.

If pain is from craning the neck on the bike:
1 Ride with a more upright posture.
2 Ride on the hoods or tops of the handlebars. Avoid the drops and use a more upright bar.
3 Reduce the distance needed to stretch. Raise or shorten the stem, use narrower handlebars and get a bike with a shorter top tube.

If pain is due to jarring:
1 Get a gel saddle.
2 Use a suspension system.
3 Ride a mountain bike on road rides.
4 Consider a recumbent.

Off-the-bicycle:
1 RICE (see p. 113).
2 Strengthening the neck muscles may help. Do not work on these muscle groups while still injured. Isometric neck exercises are helpful: use the hand to resist the motion of the head up-and-down and side-to-side. Shoulder shrugs are helpful.
3 Stretching helps some people. Voluntary range-of-motion exercises may help increase neck flexibility. Active range-of-motion exercise, with machines, weights, or forcing the neck into position, may risk injury.
4 Non-steroidal anti-inflammatory drugs (NSAIDs) are useful (see p. 114).
5 Surgery is usually the last-resort treatment. A surgical emergency may exist if the nerves being pinched in the neck interfere with muscle sensation or power elsewhere in the body.
6 Chiropractic manipulation symptomatically helps some people with pain, although many traditional physicians dispute its effectiveness.

Scapular syndrome

This is pain in the upper back, around the shoulder blade. It may or may not be associated with neck, shoulder or arm symptoms. It may or may not be related to cycling. The problem overlaps with neck ache, discussed above.

Causes

Cycling-related:
1 Extended saddle time: the longer one is in the saddle, the more time other factors act to increase tension in this area.
2 Rough terrain and jarring.
3 Too much pressure. Weight distribution too far forward puts more pressure on the upper back and neck.
4 Excessive use of upper back and neck muscles during sprinting, climbing or other efforts.

Medical. The pain may be due to a muscular problem or a pinched nerve. Cycling-related problems are due to overuse or strain. Non-cycling-related causes include pulls or strains, muscular tension related to stress or depression, arthritis and posture. If it is associated with pain that travels down the arm, is more than mild or persists for more than 2 weeks, medical attention is advised.

Treatment

On-the-bicycle:
1 Reduce mileage, readapt slowly.
2 Prevent jarring through the use of padded gloves and padded handlebar tape. Consider suspension.
3 Reduce pressure: sit more upright, vary position, raise stem height and use a shorter stem.
4 Check that the seat is not too far forward and avoid tilting the saddle down. Use a frame with a shorter top tube.
5 Avoid strain: reduce hard efforts involving the upper back muscles.

Off-the-bicycle. Avoid offending activities, including upper-body work while symptomatic, and excessive time looking at video screens.

Medical:
1 RICE: local ice may relieve the pain. If the problem relates to a pinched nerve in the neck, a neck collar may be helpful.
2 Strengthening the neck, arms and upper back may be helpful.
3 Stretching: improving neck and back flexibility may assist.
4 Massage may soothe.
5 NSAIDs are useful (see p. 114).
6 Cortisone is rarely used in this location, although injections of anesthetics, or numbing medicines, can be tried.
7 Surgery is the treatment of last resort if the cause is related to a pinched nerve.

Elbow pain

Pain either at the inside or outside of the elbow, unrelated to sudden injury, is discussed here, but injury, fracture and swelling of the elbow are not.

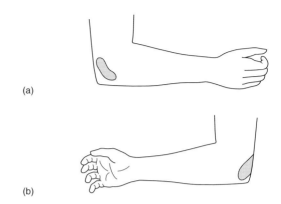

Fig. 6.1 (a) Lateral epicondylitis or 'tennis elbow'. (b) Medial epicondylitis.

Causes

Repetitive twisting usually causes the problem. The twisting irritates the forearm muscles as they rub over bony surfaces near the elbow. The irritation is often accompanied by microtears of the tendons. Pain at the outside of the elbow is lateral epicondylitis or tennis elbow (Fig. 6.1). Pain at the inside is medial epicondylitis or reverse tennis elbow. Tennis is in fact a frequent cause, but any repetitive twisting motion, whether it be polishing doorknobs, sorting items into slots, painting or shaking hands, can cause the problem.

Cycling-related elbow pain is most frequent in mountain bikers who repetitively twist gear and brake levers. It may also occur in cyclists who ride tensed-up with rigid outstretched arms.

Treatment

On-the-bicycle. Be aware of twisting motions and use a set-up that reduces the need to twist or places shifters and brakes in a more ergonometric position.

Off-the-bicycle. Avoid other offending activities.

Medical
1 RICE: a so-called tennis-elbow band or support may be helpful. These come in a variety of forms, but the key is a non-elastic strapping about 2 cm wide placed about 2 cm below the elbow. This helps stabilize the muscles that attach to the elbow. Local ice may be helpful.

2 Massage: may soothe. A special technique used in this area is friction massage.
3 Stretching: specific stretches discussed and shown may be useful.
4 NSAIDs are useful (see p. 114).
5 Cortisone may be helpful.
6 Surgery to reposition tendons is the treatment of last resort.

Cyclist's palsy (ulnar neuropathy)

This is pain, tingling, numbness and weakness in the hand along the course of the ulnar nerve. Symptoms may be present in the little and ring fingers. Symptoms are worse while riding or for several hours afterwards. Although this problem usually improves after riding stops, if it is ignored, it can lead to permanent nerve injury.

Causes

The ulnar nerve is compressed in the heel of the hand – the fleshy part of the hand below the little finger (Fig. 6.2).

Cycling-related:
1 Extended saddle time: the longer one is in the saddle, the more time other factors act to press on the hand.
2 Rough terrain causes jarring of the hands while gripping the handlebars.
3 Improper hand position: too much time on the tops with the heel of the hand pressed against the bar.
4 Too much pressure: weight distribution too far forward puts more pressure on the hands, wrists and arms.
  The affected hand is usually the one that stays on the handlebar – the one that does not reach for the water bottle.

Treatment

On-the-bicycle. Take pressure off the heel of the hand when riding. Reduce mileage and readapt slowly. Prevent jarring by using padded or gel gloves; use padded, even double, handlebar tape; and try suspension. Improve hand position: reposition the hands frequently and relax the hands, wrists and upper body. Reduce pressure. Avoid placing pressure on the heel of the hand; vary position, raise stem height, check that the seat is not too far forward, use a shorter stem, avoid tilting the saddle down, and use a shorter top tube.

Medical. NSAIDs may be helpful (see p. 114). The main thing is to reduce pressure on the heel of the hand when riding.

Carpal tunnel syndrome

This is pain, tingling, numbness and weakness in the hand along the course of the median nerve (Fig. 6.3). Symptoms may be present in the thumb, index, middle and ring fingers. Symptoms may also travel above the wrist to the elbow and shoulder and are often worse at night.

Causes

The median nerve is compressed in the wrist. Compression is usually due to inflammation. This problem is common in those who repeatedly bend their wrists at work. Grocery checkers and keyboard operators, for example, have a high incidence of this problem. It may also be associated with medical conditions such as diabetes and pregnancy.

Cycling-related
1 Extended saddle time: the longer one is in the saddle, the more time other factors act to increase

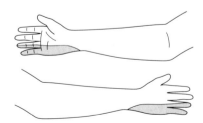

Fig. 6.2 Ulnar nerve pathway in the hand.

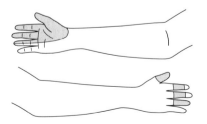

Fig. 6.3 Median nerve pathway in the hand.

inflammation in the wrist. The swelling then presses on the nerve.

2 Rough terrain: jarring of the wrists, especially while mountain biking, increases inflammation.

3 Improper wrist position: unnatural bending of the wrist while holding the handlebar predisposes to carpal tunnel syndrome.

4 Too much pressure: weight distribution too far forward places more pressure on the hands, wrists and arms.

Treatment

On-the-bicycle:

1 Reduce mileage and readapt slowly.

2 Prevent jarring by using padded gloves and padded handlebar tape. Also try suspension.

3 Improve wrist position and reposition the hands frequently. Relax the wrists and upper body. Make sure that handlebars are the correct width.

4 Reduce pressure and avoid always placing pressure on the problem wrist, using the other hand to drink from the water bottle. Vary position, raise stem height and check that the seat is not too far forward. Use a shorter stem, avoid tilting the saddle down and use a shorter top tube.

Off-the-bicycle. Reduce repetitive motion at work or elsewhere.

Medical:

1 RICE: rest in the form of wrist braces or splints is very helpful. Braces are worn at night time or around-the-clock.

2 Strengthening the wrists, arms and shoulders can help provide muscular support when riding, reducing pressure on the wrist.

3 NSAIDs are helpful (see p. 114).

4 Cortisone can be used in this location.

5 Surgery to increase the space around the nerve is common when the above methods fail.

Low back pain

This is the low backache that makes riding uncomfortable, and is pain that forces one to slow down or get off the bike. See a doctor whenever back pain is associated with loss of sensation or power in the legs. Neck pain is discussed above.

Causes of back strain

Acute low back pain can follow strain or overuse. The pain may travel to the buttock or thigh, but if nerves are not involved, it does not travel below the knee. It is usually due to:

1 muscle strain and/or spasm;

2 arthritis: usually wear-and-tear or degenerative osteoarthritis. Strain on the vertebral joints from mis-alignment, often secondary to disc degeneration, also causes pain;

3 a bulge or herniation of an intervertebral disc (discussed below).

In younger cyclists back pain is usually due to muscle strain. In older cyclists a combination of muscle strain and degenerative changes is usually responsible.

Cycling-related back strain is often related to long rides, big gears or hill work. Big-gear riding and hill climbing – especially long grades – results in back pain because riders tighten their back muscles to get more power. Position on the bike can be important. Cyclists lacking flexibility may find the aerodynamic bent-over racing position uncomfortable. Anything that forces the rider to increase stretch may cause back pain. Jarring from rough riding can be a factor.

Chronic low back pain may additionally be due to non-cycling-related factors such as: (i) leg-length difference; (ii) swayback; (iii) deconditioning and poor posture; and (iv) muscle tension caused by stress, anxiety, depression or fatigue.

Causes of nerve compression (pinched nerve)

The spinal cord travels down inside the spine or vertebral column. The vertebrae are cushioned, one from the other, by discs composed of fibre- and jelly-like material.

The spinal nerves exit between the bones of the spine, or vertebrae. Sometimes the nerves are pinched by a disc, which has been squeezed out of position between two vertebrae, or by the bones themselves.

The spinal nerves of the lower back form the sciatic nerve, which travels down the buttock area and the back of the thigh. The various component spinal nerves then travel to various parts of the leg.

Nerves have pain fibres, as well as other sensory fibres and motor or muscle-moving fibres. The progression of severity of pinched nerves is usually pain, sensory change and muscle weakness, in that order. Sensory changes include pins and needles, tingling and areas of numbness.

When a nerve is being pinched, symptoms may occur along the area supplied by the nerve. Pain radiating from the buttocks down the back of the thighs is commonly called sciatica. Pinched nerves in the back are the most frequent, but not the only cause of sciatica. Occasionally the nerve is pinched in a buttock muscle, the piriformis, rather than in the spine.

See a doctor whenever there is sensory change or muscle weakness.

Treatment

On-the-bicycle. If back strain is due to excessive exercise load:

1 Allow for a gradual increase in endurance riding. Increase the length of endurance rides no more than 10% per week.

2 If big gears are in the training programme, allow time to adapt to them slowly.

If back strain is due to hills:

1 Reduce hill mileage and then adapt to increased mileage slowly.

2 Shift positions every so often from sitting to standing. Consciously relax the back every few minutes when climbing.

3 Take a rest break at the side of the road on long climbs. Enjoy the view!

If back strain is related to an overly stretched-out position on the bike:

1 Reduce stretch by assuming a more upright posture. Ride on the hoods or tops of the handlebars.

2 Reduce the distance needed to stretch. Raise or shorten the stem. Use narrower handlebars. Get a bike with a shorter top tube.

If buttock pain or sciatica is related to nerve pressure in the piriformis muscle, get a gel-filled or more compliant saddle.

If back strain is due to jarring:

1 Get a gel saddle.

2 Use a rear suspension system.

3 Ride a mountain bike on road rides.

4 Consider a recumbent.

Off-the-bicycle:

1 RICE (see p. 113): studies show that even the worst strains do no better with bedrest beyond a few days. Mild strains may disappear as soon as one is off the bike. Ice or heat may help.

2 Strengthening the back and abdominal muscles may help. Do not work on these muscles while still injured. Gradually increasing mileage or climbing will often adapt the body sufficiently. Bent-knee sit-ups, crunches, back extensions, pelvic tilt exercises and rowing strengthen the back and abdominals.

3 Stretching helps some people. Back flexion exercises are most helpful. In individuals who have lost the normal curve (giving a flat back), extension exercises are more useful. Hamstring stretching relieves some of the need for the back to bend, and can help.

4 NSAIDs: anti-inflammatory pain medicines are useful, and are discussed on p. 114.

5 Orthotics: a heel lift or cleat shim may help if a leg-length difference exists.

6 Surgery is usually the last-resort treatment. A surgical emergency exists if the nerves being pinched interfere with bowel or bladder function, or rapidly progressive leg weakness occurs.

7 Weight loss improves back pain in many who are overweight.

8 Chiropractic manipulation symptomatically helps many with back pain, although many traditional physicians dispute its effectiveness.

Posture hints:

1 Sit or stand using a footrest to bend the knee and hip of one leg.

2 Lie either curled up on the side or on the back with pillows under the knees. Do not lie on the belly.

3 Bend from the hips and knees; avoid bending from the waist.

4 Carry or lift only what you can handle with ease.

5 Turn and face the object you wish to lift.

6 Hold heavy objects close to the body.

7 Avoid lifting heavy objects higher than the waist.

8 Avoid carrying unbalanced loads.

9 Avoid sudden movements.

10 Change positions frequently.

11 Work with tools close to the body. Avoid long reaches when raking, hoeing, mopping or vacuuming.

12 Sit down to dress. Bend the leg when putting on shoes and socks; do not bend from the waist.

13 Wear low heels.

Saddle sores

Sores of the buttocks and groin area are a common occupational hazard for the bicycle rider. Many causes can be avoided. Specific treatment is available if saddle sores do develop. The phrase 'saddle sores' is used by different riders to refer to a number of different problems involving the skin of the upper thigh and of the rear end:

1 Furuncles and folliculitis: blocked and/or infected glands and lumps are a common cycling problem. These painful bumps are classic saddle sores.

2 Ischial tuberosity pain: this is pain in the area of the pelvic bones that bear the weight on the bicycle seat. The ischial tuberosities are the 'sitting bones'. Occasionally, pain in this area progresses to either local bursitis or ulceration.

3 Chafing of the thigh: chafing of the inside of the upper leg is common in cyclists. It occurs because of friction caused by repeated rubbing of the inside of the thigh during the up-and-down motion of the pedal stroke. Many cyclists note that the inside of their shorts pills and wears with friction. When this happens to the inner thighs, redness and discomfort are the results. Dampness of the cycling shorts related to sweat production and the lack of breathability of the shorts material may make the problem worse.

4 Skin ulceration: skin that is missing its topmost surface layers and is denuded is ulcerated. This is sometimes an extreme result of rubbing or pressure.

5 Subcutaneous nodules: these are a specific type of lump found in high-mileage male cyclists near the scrotum, sometimes called 'extra testicles'.

6 Tailbone abscess: a genetic predisposition to a blocked pilonidal sinus may be aggravated by cycling and become infected. Surgical treatment is often advised.

Causes

Infection, pressure and friction are the three main causes of saddle sores. Classic saddle sores have two prevalent theories behind their origin.

The first refers to infection and blocked glands. Bacteria enter the glands, causing saddle sores. Therefore, treatment is directed at reducing the level of skin bacteria and preventing pore blockage.

The second theory is connected with pressure and friction. According to this theory, increased saddle pressure (which often arises through increased mileage) prevents small blood vessels from bringing blood to the skin and the skin receives fewer nutrients. This causes a breakdown in the skin's defences, pore irritation and blockage. Trapped bacteria may proliferate and a saddle sore develops.

Riders who always have saddle sores on the same cheek may find that their leg on that side is shorter. The buttock of a shorter leg is subject to more bumping and bruising.

Prevention

1 Keep dry. Modern synthetics wick away moisture and are softer on the skin than traditional leather chamois. Do not continue to wear wet sweat-drenched shorts after riding. Change into loose shorts that allow air to circulate. After bathing, allow the crotch to dry completely before putting on tight-fitting shorts or cycling shorts. Powder in the shorts can prevent chafing that may lead to irritation and infected blocked glands (although powder may be linked to some cervical problems in women).

2 Keep clean.

3 Wear synthetic padded cycling shorts.

4 Always wear clean cycling shorts. Avoid wearing the same shorts 2 days in a row without laundering. Soiled shorts not only have more bacteria, they do not breathe as well as freshly laundered ones.

5 Avoid cycling shorts that are pilled or with seams in areas that rub the inside thigh or on which pressure is placed.

6 Do not suddenly and drastically increase weekly mileage.

7 Use seats that provide enough padding or support and spread the support over as wide an area as is compatible with the anatomy.

8 Check seat position.

9 Avoid shaving from above the short line to the groin. This often results in red spots, caused by irritation and infection.

Treatment

Self-treatment:

1 Apply all the preventive measures described above.

2 Modify training. One may need to reduce training, or climb more out of the saddle.

3 Soak in a comfortably hot bath three times a day for 15 min to allow boils to come to the surface and drain. Hot-water soaks increase blood circulation to the inflamed area, allowing more of the body's healing factors access to the area.

4 For classic saddle sores or ischial tuberosity pain, pad the skin with padded tape or moleskin. One may want to reduce the tackiness of moleskin by first applying it to something other than the skin. Leave some tack so that it will still stick, but not so much that it pulls the skin and hair off when removed later.

5 Another possibility is to take a couple of adhesive plasters or a layer of moleskin and cut out a small hole for the sore, effectively padding around the sore and taking pressure off the sore itself.

6 The extra padding of a second pair of shorts worn over the first may help.

7 A padded seat cover may improve the situation.

8 A different seat may resolve the problem.

9 Suspension may help. Rear-end suspension or beamed seat tubes reduce saddle pressure.

10 A modification of seat position – nose up or down, forward or back, up or down – may help.

11 Friction-related problems may be helped by an emollient, such as petroleum jelly (Vaseline).

12 Topical cortisone, antifungal and antibacterial creams may help.

13 Some riders swear by a veterinary product called 8-hydroxyguinoline sulfate in petroleum and lanolin.

14 Shimming the shoe of the shorter leg may help if saddle sores are related to leg-length discrepancy.

Medical and surgical:

1 If the area around the sore is infected, it may require surgical drainage or antibiotics.

2 Uninfected sores that remain painful, swollen or with hard lumps can occasionally be treated with a cortisone injection.

3 Occasionally, surgery may be required to remove chronic cysts.

Haemorrhoids

Symptomatic haemorrhoids are painful or itchy varicose veins at the end of the gastrointestinal tract – the anus. They may also bleed. They may be internal or external. The painful ones are usually caused by a blood clot in an external haemorrhoid.

Causes

Haemorrhoids are associated with prolonged sitting, constipation and pregnancy. It is uncertain whether cycling causes haemorrhoids, but saddle-sitting can certainly make them noticeable and uncomfortable.

Treatment

Most painful external haemorrhoids improve on their own. Hot (not burning) tub soaks may help. Creams may help ease irritation, but are useless for pain. If one cannot sit down, simple surgical excision removes the clot and eases pain.

Crotch dermatitis

Crotch dermatitis or crotchitis is irritation or inflammation of the crotch. Redness, itching and pain are problems in this area. Crotchitis is common in women – specifically, irritation of the skin around the vagina, the clitoris and the urethra. Crotchitis is distinctive from saddle sores, discussed above. The best treatment is prevention. Some general measures help almost all cases of crotchitis. Some treatments may improve some causes of crotchitis, but may make other cases worse. It is therefore important to determine the cause of crotchitis.

Causes

Many cases of crotchitis are related to a combination of factors.

1 Warmth and moisture aggravate most cases of crotchitis. Avoid travelling to races or rides already wearing bike shorts and only change into bike shorts on arrival. Use bike shorts with a breathable, moisture-wicking crotch. Change out of moist or wet cycling shorts as soon as possible after riding. Wear loose-fitting shorts or a skirt. Wear breathable fabrics and cotton underwear. Avoid tight-fitting non-breathing underwear, or wear no underwear. Pantyhose is an enemy of the crotch.

Allow ventilation to cool and dry the area. Avoid sitting on non-breathing surfaces such as plastic and leather. Use a car-seat cover with air holes if the car has vinyl or leather seats.

Moisture and warmth cause yeast overgrowth, commonly called jock itch or crotch rot. Over-the-counter antifungal creams and powders may help reduce yeast overgrowth. Occasionally irritated skin can also be helped by over-the-counter cortisone cream, although cortisone sometimes worsens yeast overgrowth.

2 Hygiene and irritants. Stool is a powerful irritant so clean properly. Overzealous hygiene can be as much of a problem as lack of hygiene. With irritation, wiping and rubbing can cause chafing and further irritation. Since this area always has some bacteria, and since irritated skin is prone to worsen and become infected, overzealous wiping must be avoided. Avoid wiping affected areas with rough toilet tissue.

Wipe the anal area from front to back. Women need to avoid carrying bacteria towards the vagina and urethra. Not only is crotchitis worsened, but urinary tract infections and vaginal infections may result.

Avoid local irritants such as harsh soaps. If crotchitis extends to areas which need to be wiped to keep clean, consider using facial tissue, gentle medicated over-the-counter products such as Tucks (witch-hazel pads), moistened toilet paper or plain water. Clean, and then pat – not wipe – dry.

3 Friction. Friction can be minimized by using an emollient skin preparation, such as petroleum jelly or an antiyeast cream. A seat pad or cover fitted over the saddle may allow slight movement and function, similar to how a sock protects in a shoe.

Wearing two pairs of light-weight bicycling shorts or a light-weight bicycling liner may help reduce friction-caused crotchitis. But if crotchitis is related to warmth and moisture, doubling up on shorts may make things worse.

4 Bicycle position and saddle. Most bicycles are sold for men, and the top tube stem length results in too much reach for most women. This puts extra pressure on the crotch. Make sure the bicycle position is not too stretched out.

Saddle position and type may be factors relating to crotchitis. Consider seat angle. Nose-down slightly may help, especially for time-trial events or crits where one is in an aerodynamic position and putting substantial pressure on the crotch. Some women prefer a nose-up position so that the saddle presses more on the pubic bone and less on the soft tissues around the vagina.

Move around frequently. Get off that saddle when possible. Stand up on the pedals to relieve crotch friction and pressure. Climb hills standing up periodically. When descending, put weight on the pedals to relieve the crotch. This allows moving air to cool and dry the crotch while easing pressure. If riding tandem, be sure to take frequent crotch breaks by getting out of the saddle at stop signs and stop lights and by standing at least every 15 min.

American-made Terry saddles have padding and are less stiff. Many women report that, although they feel no different from other saddles while riding, at the end of a ride their crotch does not hurt as much. Extreme cases of crotchitis may require drastic measures: cutting or paring the seat may be necessary to keep riding.

5 Allergies. Many riders use a wide variety of products in this area that may cause allergies. To help with saddle sores near the crotch, riders may use tapes or pads to which they may have a tape allergy. This may induce crotchitis. Some riders use perfumed or chemically treated products, including sprays, sanitary napkins or lubricating oils, to which they may be allergic. These can then cause or worsen crotchitis.

6 Vaginal infections. The extra moisture related to a vaginal infection may worsen crotchitis. Treating the underlying vaginal discharge may help improve the condition. Infected or otherwise blocked sweat or other glands may develop into crotchitis if friction worsens these conditions.

7 Other infections. Occasionally other infections, such as herpes, cause crotch irritation. Crotch irritation can also promote or eacerbate herpes outbreaks in people who harbour the virus.

8 Medical problems. Riders with skin conditions such as psoriasis or eczema may have flare-ups in this areas related to friction and other general factors, listed above. Prescription-strength cortisone creams are often the best help for this. Occasionally, other medical problems such as lactose intolerance or pinworms are the cause.

Knees: introduction

Overuse knee problems related to the repeated and constant stresses of riding over time are one of the most frequent reasons cyclists seek medical advice.

Table 6.1 Bicycle adjustment based on the location of knee pain.

Location	Causes	Solutions
Anterior	Seat too low	Raise seat
	Seat too far forward	Move seat back
	Climbing too much	Reduce climbing
	Big gears, low rpm	Spin more
	Cranks too long	Shorten cranks
Medial	Cleats: toes point out	Modify cleat position: toe in
		Consider floating pedals
	Floating pedals	Limit float to 5°
	Exiting clipless pedals	Lower tension
	Feet too far apart	Modify cleat position: move closer
		Shorten bottom bracket axle
		Use cranks with less offset
Lateral	Cleats: toes point in	Modify cleat: toe out
		Consider floating pedals
	Floating pedals	Limit float to 5°
	Feet too close	Modify cleat position: apart
		Longer bottom bracket axle
		Use cranks with more offset
		Shim pedal on crank 2 mm
Posterior	Saddle too high	Lower saddle
	Saddle too far back	Move saddle forward
	Floating pedals	Limit float to 5°

Some knee problems are sudden injuries related to trauma – a bicycle crash, or the sudden tearing of a cartilage or ligament. Sudden injuries, injuries with significant local swelling (water on the knee), knee clicking, knee instability and knee collapse are not discussed here. Torn ligaments, torn menisci and fractures generally require prompt professional medical attention.

Significant local redness or warmth may indicate an infection and requires prompt medical attention. Those with a history of gout or other forms of arthritis are advised to seek medical attention. The different kinds of knee arthritis are not discussed in this book.

Mild problems may be self-treated, but any problem that does not respond within a couple of weeks is deserving of expert advice.

Knee complaints can usually be identified as anterior (in the front), medial (inside), lateral (outside) or posterior (back) of the knee. The discussion of specific knee problems will follow this organization. Even without knowing the diagnosis, by knowing where the knee hurts it is possible to make bicycle-position recommendations (Table 6.1).

Chondromalacia patellae

The kneecap, or patella, is in front of the knee (Fig. 6.4). It glides over the end of the thigh bone, or femur. Sometimes the underside surface of the kneecap is roughened, or softened, and instead of gliding smoothly it rubs roughly over the end of the

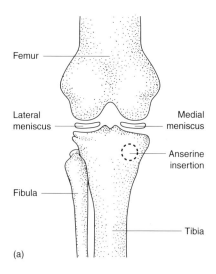

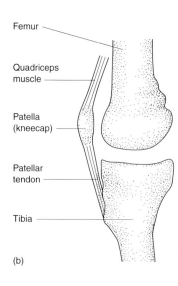

Fig. 6.4 (a) Front view of the knee (patella and quadriceps removed). (b) Side view of the knee.

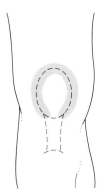

Fig. 6.5 Front of the knee tenderness. Tenderness here is usually due to chondromalacia or arthritis.

thigh bone. This problem is sometimes called patellofemoral dysfunction, or patellofemoral syndrome, because of the anatomical location of this problem.

A grating sensation at the front of the knee (Fig. 6.5), pain when walking down stairs and a general ache are frequent features. Stiffness after prolonged seating (movie-goer's stiffness) is common.

Causes

The kneecap is not flat on its underside, but has a ridge. As the knee bends, this ridge follows a path along the surface of the thigh bone. Excessive force pushing the kneecap on to the surface of the end of the thigh bone creates excessive stress – called loading or shearing force – on the underside of the kneecap and may result in its surface becoming roughened. Some individuals are genetically predisposed to a rough kneecap.

Some of the bicycling causes of excessive loading or shearing forces are hill climbing and big-gear time trialling. Weight training, running, squatting, kneeling and climbing also place increased pressure on the patellofemoral surface.

A muscle or posture imbalance may cause the knee-cap to stray from its ideal path over the surface of the femur. When not gliding over its ideal path, the patella is subject to increased forces and becomes roughened. A relative weakness of the medial (inside aspect of the leg) quadriceps muscle is often

responsible. A wide pelvis and 'knock knees' may make the condition more likely.

This tends to be an early-season injury.

Treatment

On-the-bicycle. Bicycling correctly often helps this problem. Many runners suffer from chondromalacia, and bicycle riding is often suggested for therapy. A roughened kneecap will often smooth out over time if offending activities are stopped.

A relatively high-in-the-saddle position helps – with the knee bent not more than 25° from horizontal when the foot is at the bottom of the stroke. Sitting farther back in the saddle helps. Spinning rather than big gears (a cadence of 85 rpm or more) helps. Avoid hills, and especially long climbs. Stand more when climbing. Avoid long cranks.

If due to a tracking problem, rather than a load problem, pedals allowing some free rotation may help.

Off-the-bicycle. Weight-lifting machines usually increase the load or shearing forces of the patella on the femur. Exercises where the knee is bent more than 90° place increased loads on these surfaces and may worsen the problem. Squats, leg presses and leg extensions all place increased loads on the patellofemoral surface.

Avoid squatting, kneeling, walking or running downstairs. Avoid running at all. Above all, avoid running down hills.

Medical:
1 RICE (see p. 113).
2 Strengthening the medial quadriceps may help. Look for exercises that involve only the last part of straightening the leg (terminal extension exercises). Remember to be cautious about strength training when injured. Use strength training primarily to prevent reinjury. Machines that limit the bend in the knee to 15–20° from straight-out, and then allow completion of the last 15–20° of extension, are helpful.

Try placing a couple of pillows under the knee, while lying down. With weight around the ankle, lift and straighten the knee, and hold for a couple of seconds, then relax. Repeat up to 100 times. Athletes may use weights up to about one-quarter of body weight. Elite cyclists may have difficulty placing enough weight on their ankle to make this exercise worthwhile.

Step-ups to a height of one step may be helpful. With only body weight at first, face a 20–25 cm step, and place the foot of the affected leg on the step. Raise up. Lower. Repeat 15–20 times. As balance is developed, hold weights in the hands or place a barbell on the back. Elite cyclists may lift up to their own body weight in barbell load.

Isometric exercises with the leg outstretched and no change in position during the exercise may be helpful. Since this exercise can be performed in any position – standing, sitting or lying – it is easy to perform hundreds of 20–30 s repetitions daily.

3 Stretching: quadriceps exercises are particularly useful (see p. 114).
4 NSAIDs are discussed on p. 114.
5 Orthotics: if excessive foot pronation results in under-the-kneecap discomfort, orthotics may help.
6 Cortisone is not used in this location.
7 Surgery is the treatment of last resort. The underside of the roughened kneecap may be smoothed. If the gliding path of the kneecap is incorrect, repositioning tendons may be tried. This is a drastic step.

Patellar tendinitis

The patellar tendon attaches the bottom of the patella to the tibial tubercle, a prominence on the front top of the shin bone. As with other tendons, inflammation or irritation in this area results in tendinitis. This type of tendinitis may take a relatively long time to resolve with continued riding.

A specific variant of this problem is mostly found in adolescent boys – Osgood–Schlatter disease. Here pain is found where the patellar tendon attaches to the shin bone (Fig. 6.6).

Causes

Tendinitis in this area from repetitive bicycling stress may follow a one-time injury to this area, or result from poor bike fit. Low saddle, forward position, big gears and long hills all contribute to this problem.

Some people's anatomy tends to predispose them to this condition.

In Osgood–Schlatter disease, growth of the bones during the growth spurt results in a pulling at the

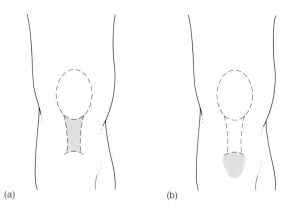

Fig. 6.6 Front of the knee tenderness. (a) Tenderness here is usually due to patellar tendinitis. (b) Tenderness here is usually due to Osgood–Schlatter disease.

attachment of the patellar tendon at the tibial tubercle – the forward top prominence of the shin bone.

Tenderness at the lower edge of the kneecap is occasionally due to a stress fracture.

Treatment

On-the-bicycle. A relatively high-in-the-saddle position helps. Make sure that the knee is not bent more than 25° from horizontal when the foot is at the bottom of the stroke. A position farther back in the saddle helps. Spin rather than use big gears and maintain a cadence of 85 rpm or more. Avoid hills, and especially long climbs. Avoid long cranks. Limit flotation to 5°.

Off-the-bicycle. The same recommendations apply as for chondromalacia above. Jumping sports are particularly associated with patellar tendinitis.

Medical. See chondromalacia patellae, above.
1 RICE, discussed on p. 113, may be helpful.
2 Stretching quadriceps exercises are useful.
3 Orthotics can help.
4 NSAIDs are discussed on p. 114.
5 Cortisone is not used in this location.
6 Surgery is not used in this location.

Quadriceps tendinitis

The quadriceps tendons attach the ends of the quadriceps muscles to either the upper pole of the patella or the shin bone. Like other tendons, inflammation or irritation in this area results in tendinitis. This type of tendinitis may take a relatively long time to resolve with continued riding.

Causes

Tendinitis in this area from repetitive bicycling stress may follow a one-time injury to this area, or result from poor bike fit. Low saddle, forward position, big gears and long hills all contribute to this problem.

Treatment

Treatment is the same as for patellar tendinitis and chondromalacia above, unless the medial quadriceps is involved, in which case terminal extension exercises are to be avoided as well.

Prepatellar bursitis

Prepatellar bursitis involves swelling and perhaps some discomfort over the lower kneecap and patellar tendon caused by a swelling of the covering envelope, or bursa. If this area is red, warm or tender, it may be necessary to aspirate the bursa to make sure it is not infected.

Causes

Overuse irritation from frequent prolonged kneeling, such as seen in carpet-layer's or floor-scrubbing housemaid's knee, is also common. Continued irritation from an initial injury, such as a fall, occurs in cyclists.

Treatment

Off-the-bicycle. Avoid kneeling or use knee pads if kneeling must be continued. The treatment is the same as for patellar tendinitis and chondromalacia, above.

Medical
1 NSAIDs are discussed on p. 114.
2 Cortisone has a fair success rate, together with fluid drainage.
3 Surgery may remove a chronically inflamed bursa.

Arthritis of the knee

Many forms of knee arthritis exist. The most common,

osteoarthritis or degenerative joint disease, occurs as we age. It is simply the wear and tear of the joint. A pain or ache is felt in the front of the knee, or throughout the knee.

Causes

The cause is wear and tear from ageing. The additional knee stress of obesity, pushing big gears, or of climbing may also contribute.

Treatment

Basically, the treatment is the same as for chondromalacia, above.
1 NSAIDs are a mainstay of treatment (see p. 114).
2 Cortisone is occasionally used.
3 Surgery, including total knee replacement, is used in the most severe cases.

Anserine tendinitis

The anserine tendon attaches at the upper inner aspect of the shin bone (Fig. 6.7). It is really the coming together of three muscles – the semitendinosus, gracilis and sartorius. This tendon, or its bursa underneath, becomes irritated and inflamed.

Causes

The cause is increased pressure of the medial knee. Extra force is caused by having the toes pointed outwards or the knees too far apart when cycling. Exiting clipless pedals stresses the ligaments and tendons of

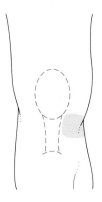

Fig. 6.7 Medial knee tenderness (right knee). Tenderness here is often due to anserine tendinitis.

the medial knee. Occasionally, improper saddle position is a factor.

Some people's anatomy tends to predispose to this condition – those with turned-in shin bones, pronation and bowed legs.

Treatment

On-the-bicycle. If fixed cleats are used, adjust them so that the toes point slightly more inward. If floating pedals are used, limit flotation to 5°. Reduce the tension of clipless pedals to allow easier exit. Reduce the distance between the feet by: (i) positioning the cleat so that the foot is closer to the crank, (ii) using a narrower bottom bracket axle, or (iii) using cranks with less offset. Use a proper saddle position and spin over 85 rpm. Reduce mileage.

Off-the-bicycle. Avoid running on inclines, especially when the affected leg is on the uphill side. Roller blading and skiing may make this problem worse.

Medical:
1 RICE, discussed on p. 113, is useful.
2 Stretching is an important therapy.
3 NSAIDs are useful (see p. 114).
4 Orthotics may help.
5 Cortisone is used.
6 Surgery is rarely used and is a last resort.

Plica (patellofemoral ligament inflammation)

A plica is a fold or thickened band of tissue. Arising within the knee, it causes discomfort most frequently in the medial aspect of the knee. An inflamed medial patellofemoral ligament (a ligament between the kneecap and the thigh bone) causes similar symptoms. A torn medial meniscus (cartilage) also causes similar symptoms. Often, only surgery will enable the correct diagnosis to be made.

Pain often occurs within a reproducible range of motion – once on the downstroke, once on the upstroke. If locking or swelling of the knee is present, consult an orthopaedist or sports-medicine physician.

Causes

Increased pressure on the inside of the knee is related

to the problem. Extra force is caused by having the toes pointed outward or the knees too far apart when cycling. Occasionally, improper saddle position is a factor.

Some people's anatomy tends to predispose to this condition – those with turned-in shin bones, pronation or bowed legs.

Treatment

On-the-bicycle. If fixed cleats are used, adjust them so that the toes point slightly more inward. If floating pedals are used, limit flotation to 5°. Reduce the distance between the feet by: (i) positioning the cleat so that the foot is closer to the crank, (ii) using a narrower bottom bracket axle, or (iii) using cranks with less offset. Use a proper saddle position and spin over 85 rpm. Reduce mileage.

Off-the-bicycle. Cyclists have this problem as often as other athletes. Running, skiing and roller blading make the problem worse.

Medical:
1 RICE is discussed on p. 113.
2 Stretching may help.
3 NSAIDs are discussed on p. 114.
4 Orthotics may help.
5 Cortisone is not used.
6 Surgery may be necessary to differentiate medial plica, medial patellofemoral ligament and medial meniscal problems. Knee locking and repeated knee swelling may indicate the need for surgery.

Iliotibial band syndrome

The iliotibial band is a fibrous band of tissue running along the lateral knee. It rubs over the lateral surface of the knee, especially when the knee is bent about 30°. It is commonly inflamed, causing pain in this area (Fig. 6.8).

Causes

Excessive stretch on this area is the most common cause. It results from too much pull on the lateral knee. Maladjusted cleat position, with the toes pointing in, is the most frequent cause. A narrow

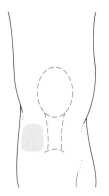

Fig. 6.8 Lateral knee tenderness (right knee). Tenderness here is often due to iliotibial band tendinitis.

bottom bracket or cranks with little offset may be associated with iliotibial band syndrome. Low saddle height and excessive forces due to big gears and hills are contributing factors.

Sometimes iliotibial band syndrome develops after a fall and a bruise to this area.

Some people's anatomy tends to predispose to this condition, especially those with a wide pelvis. Tight gluteal muscles can be a contributing factor.

Treatment

On-the-bicycle. Readjust the cleats to allow the toes to point out slightly more. Limit flotation to 5°. Increase the distance between the feet by (i) positioning the cleats so that the foot is farther from the crank, (ii) inserting a 2 mm spacer between the pedal and the crank, (iii) using a wider bottom bracket, or (iv) using cranks with more offset. Reduce hill work. A floating pedal system may help. Make sure the saddle height is not too low or too high, and not too far back.

Off-the-bicycle. Avoid running, especially across inclines where the affected leg is uphill.

Medical:
1 RICE is discussed on p. 113.
2 Strengthening side kicks and slide board exercise may either help or worsen this problem.
3 Stretching: specific stretches are discussed.
4 Orthotics can help.
5 NSAIDs are discussed on p. 114.

6 Cortisone can be used if other methods fail.
7 Surgery is a last resort.

Tight hamstrings

The muscles in the back of the thigh are known as the hamstrings. Tightness in this area is a common cause of pain behind the knee.

Causes

High seat position and sitting too far back in the saddle are contributing factors. Dropping the heel when climbing and pushing big gears worsen the problem. Lack of flexibility is usually present.

Improper cleat position can be a factor in fixed-pedal systems. Sometimes excessive pedal float is related to this problem because the hamstrings help to stabilize the leg when pedalling.

Relative weakness of the hamstrings, compared to the strength of the quads, can be a contributing factor.

Treatment

On-the-bicycle. Sit further forward in the saddle. Avoid a high saddle position. Avoid dropping the heels when pushing a big gear or climbing. Use pedals which limit float to less than 5°.

Medical:
1 RICE, discussed on p. 113, is useful.
2 Strengthening: tight hamstrings are often weak hamstrings. Strengthening exercises are useful.
3 Stretching is the most important therapy.
4 NSAIDs are discussed on p. 114.
5 Orthotics rarely help.
6 Cortisone is not used.
7 Surgery is rarely used and is a last resort.

Baker's cyst

A Baker's cyst is found behind the knee. It is a swelling of a sac that either has its origins within the knee or from a bursa associated with a muscle behind the knee. It is an occasional cause of pain behind the knee. If the cyst ruptures, it can cause calf pain which may mimic the pain of a blood clot.

Causes

Baker's cyst is caused by a weakness in the tissues. When associated with a sac that has its origins within the knee, it often indicates a more serious problem within the knee.

Treatment

On-the-bicycle. Sit further forward in the saddle. Avoid a high saddle position. Avoid dropping the heels when pushing a big gear or climbing.

Medical:
1 RICE is discussed on p. 113.
2 Stretching will probably not help.
3 NSAIDs are discussed on p. 114.
4 Orthotics do not help.
5 Cortisone is not used.
6 Surgery is frequently helpful in removing the cyst and curing the problem. It may also be helpful to correct any related internal knee problems.

Tibialis anterior tendinitis

This is inflammation of the shin muscles. Shin splints, or anterior lower-leg pain, is much more common in runners.

Causes

The cause is excessive tendon strain on the upstroke, especially when the foot is dorsiflexed, or bent upward.

Treatment

On-the-bicycle. Avoid a forceful pull-up. Occasionally, a high saddle contributes to the problem. Lowering the saddle may help.

Off-the bicycle. Avoid running, especially on hills.

Medical:
1 RICE is discussed on p. 113.
2 NSAIDs are discussed on p. 114.

Achilles tendinitis

This is inflammation of the Achilles tendon, the giant tendon at the back of the foot, at the bottom of the back of the leg. A different problem in this area is bursitis (see below). For pain at the bottom of the heel, see the section on heel pain syndrome (below).

Problems in this area are not unusual in cyclists, but occur less frequently than knee overuse problems.

Causes

Excessive stretch from unaccustomed activity usually causes the problem. This most often results from a new shoe or cleat, especially when the net consequence is that extension of the leg has been increased. For example, if a rider is used to the Shimano clipless system and changes to Speedplay, the shoe–pedal distance is reduced. This means that it is necessary to lower the seat. If this is not done, excess stretch occurs and the rider is at risk for Achilles tendinitis.

Somewhat paradoxically, a seat that is too low can also cause Achilles tendinitis. In an attempt to generate more power, the rider may drop the back of the foot, placing excessive and repeated stretch on the Achilles tendon.

With unequal leg lengths, the shorter leg is more likely to have an Achilles problem. A cleat too far forward or positioned so that the foot is toed-in occasionally causes this problem. Soft or flexible soles may contribute. Cold, wet-weather riding, where the back of the sock becomes wet and cold, may cause the problem.

Treatment

On-the-bicycle. Ride if pain free. Hills are usually harder on the Achilles tendon, so reduce hill mileage.

Off-the-bicycle. If associated with another activity, that activity may need to be modified. For example, if Achilles tendinitis is associated with new shoes with a lower heel used for walking or running, a heel pad or lift may help.

Medical:
1 RICE: rest and hot or cold compresses may be helpful (see p. 113).
2 Stretching is important once the problem improves, but not while it is still painful. Until improved reduce the stretch on the Achilles tendon. For most riders, this means lowering the saddle a few millimetres.

3 Orthotics can help.
4 NSAIDs may be helpful (see p. 114).
5 Cortisone should never be used. It weakens the tendon and may cause rupture.
6 Surgery is a last resort.

Achilles bursitis

This is commonly called a pump bump; another medical name is posterior calcaneal bursitis. It is caused by the heel counter of a shoe irritating the bursa. It is best to avoid the offending shoe, or cut out the relevant heel counter.

Medical treatment

1 RICE: hot or cold compresses may be helpful (see p. 113).
2 NSAIDs may help (see p. 113).
3 Cortisone is occasionally helpful. Avoid a cortisone injection if the problem is tendinitis: it weakens the tendon and may cause a rupture.
4 Surgery is a last resort.

Heel pain syndrome (plantar fasciitis)

This is pain at the bottom of the heel. For pain on the back of the heel, see Achilles tendinitis (above). The plantar fascia is a fibrous band in the foot arch that runs from the toes to the heel. It helps support the arch and prevents it from collapsing. Inflammation of this band, or plantar fasciitis, is the usual cause of pain in this area.

Sometimes a bone spur, or pointed growth of bone, develops where the foot ligaments attach to the heel, or calcaneus bone, and is associated with this problem.

Causes

Inflammation occurs where the plantar fascia attaches to the heel due to excessive repetitive stretch from chronic foot strain. Excessive pronation and a low-arched or high-arched foot are common causes. The immediate cause is often not related to cycling. But many things cyclists do, such as running and weight lifting, are associated with the problem. It may also be related to non-cycling shoes that are too stiff-soled, being overweight, hiking or carrying heavy loads.

An X-ray may or may not show a spur. Usually the spur is an indication of a long-term problem; it is not itself the cause of the pain.

Medical treatment

1 RICE is discussed on p. 113. Icing for 10 min twice a day may help.
2 Strengthening: foot exercises may be helpful; for example: (i) walk on the outsides of bare feet 10 min twice a day, and (ii) with the foot bare, use the toes to grab hold of and lift up a face cloth. Hold for a count of five and then let go. Build up to 20 times twice a day.
3 Stretching: facing a wall, with the foot planted about 1 m from the wall, lean against the wall with the leg straight. Repeat with the knee bent. A pull should be felt in the calf. Increasing the flexibility of the Achilles tendon reduces the need for this area to stretch and reduces strain on the plantar fascia.
4 Orthotics may help. A heel pad or waffle support, also known as a tulle cup, may help.
5 NSAIDs: anti-inflammatory pain medicines are useful and are discussed on p. 114.
6 Cortisone: a local steroid injection has a fair success rate.
7 Surgery is usually the treatment of last resort.

Foot or toe numbness (hot and cold foot)

This is pain, burning or numbness in the ball of the feet or the toes. In cool weather, the foot may be cold.

Causes

Pain, burning and numbness is almost always caused by pressure around the foot. Old-style cleats with toe straps that are too tight, shoes that are too tight, or shoe straps cinched too tightly are the usual causes. Occasionally, high mileage and an improperly posi-tioned cleat contribute to the problem. Sometimes the cause is arthritis or a non-cycling-related medical condition.

In cool weather, cold feet may result from compression of the foot and a resulting decrease in blood circulation.

Treatment

For pain, burning or numbness, the solution is to relieve the pressure. Loosen the toe straps, loosen the shoes, and buy wider or larger shoes. When stopping for lunch or rest, even if only for a few minutes, take off the shoes and wiggle the toes.

Occasionally the problem relates to cleat position. Usually the cleat needs to be placed further back, although solutions differ. Do whatever allows the foot more room in the shoe. An irregularity of the sole – sometimes a manufacturing defect – may press on the ball of the foot. Look for cleat bolts that are pushing through the sole, causing it to be uneven. Too much or too little cleat–shoe contact may contribute to the problem. Orthotics, which can spread the pressure, may help.

Occasionally the problem relates to a swollen nerve – a Morton's neuroma. Local cortisone, orthotics or surgical removal of the neuroma are options.

For cold feet, relieve the pressure, consider wider or larger shoes that allow room for thermal socks, or use shoe covers.

Traumatic injuries

Some traumatic or sudden injuries occur in cycling with increased frequency. Other injuries are associated with cycling-specific treatments which allow athletes to return to riding sooner. Traumatic injuries are discussed in general first, including sprains and strains, and the initial management of a potentially serious accident is then considered.

Specific traumatic injuries, such as abrasions, collarbone fracture and shoulder separation, are covered because of their frequency in cyclists or because of their cycling-specific treatment. Serious head injury is not a common injury, and treatment in cyclists follows the same lines as in other individuals. Because head injuries are potentially fatal, and are often preventable with the use of helmets, this topic will also be discussed.

This section is not meant to be a comprehensive review of all traumatic injuries in cycling. Injuries that do occur in cyclists, but with low frequency or which are treated in the same way as in non-cyclists, such as splenic rupture or carpal bone fracture, will not be discussed.

General anatomical classification

Traumatic injuries commonly affect ligaments (sprains and dislocations), tendons or muscles (strains), the skin (abrasions and lacerations), bones (fractures) and internal organs (contusions and lacerations).

A *sprain* is a stretching injury to a ligament or group of ligaments. First-degree sprains involve only excessive stretching, second-degree sprains are partial tears and third-degree sprains are complete tears of ligaments. On examination, first-degree sprains have no abnormal laxity (looseness of the joint), while third-degree sprains have no end-point (the ligament is not holding the joint together).

Stress X-rays are often obtained to determine the severity of sprains. However, many dispute their relevance, feeling that clinical examination is at least as accurate. In an immature skeleton, an apparent sprain may be a fracture through a growth plate. Although stress radiographs may confirm the diagnosis, manipulation may worsen the injury.

Third-degree sprains almost always require orthopaedic consultation.

A *strain* is an injury to muscle or tendon. Often considered to be a stretching injury, strains may also result from inappropriate internal tension, which is a slightly different concept. Some think that avulsion-type fracture is a type of strain. First-degree strains only involve excessive stretching, second-degree strains are partial tears, while third-degree strains are complete tears. In young adults these injuries usual occur at the muscle–tendon junction; in older individuals the tendon itself is usually the site of injury.

First-degree strains often occur over a series of muscle motions. The athlete may notice a pop or snap with a single motion, signifying a second-degree strain. The dramatic pop or snap of a third-degree strain is often heard by others.

Basic field management

Fractures, limb- and life-threatening injuries occasionally occur in cycling. These situations often create chaos and confusion. An apparent injury is often not the one most in need of attention. Here are some basic steps for immediately dealing with a severe injury.

1 Prevent further injury to the rider and others. Are there other immediate hazards? Are others hurt? Evaluate the overall risks of the scene of the accident before attending to the fallen rider. Establish whether the rider has fallen in a relatively safe location, or

whether the location presents an immoderate risk to him- or herself or others, in which case the rider must be moved immediately.

Ask one or two others to act as traffic control, keeping traffic from running over the rider and preventing further injuries. Remove other riders and spectators from the roadway, except for those providing necessary assistance.

2 Is the rider breathing well? If the rider is not breathing, cardiopulmonary resuscitation may be necessary. If the rider is having trouble breathing, a significant chest injury may be present. If he or she is breathing normally, talking or cursing, there is usually no need to do anything for at least several minutes. It will take at least several minutes after a fall for a rider to gather his or her wits and be ready to converse intelligently and answer questions.

3 Is neck pain present? Is there movement in both arms and legs? If the rider has neck pain or cannot move some part of the extremities he or she may have a serious neck or spinal injury and should not be moved.

If the rider has no neck pain and can move the arms and legs, and wishes to move, that is fine. Never move a rider who does not want to move unless there is a serious risk of further injury (for example, because of being in the middle of a heavy traffic lane).

4 Is arterial bleeding present? Bright red spurting blood signals arterial bleeding. Apply and maintain direct pressure to stop the bleeding.

5 Can the rider sit and stand up? If the rider is unable to sit and stand up alone, after a few minutes to catch the breath, he or she probably needs an ambulance.

6 Call for help. If the rider needs an ambulance, call the country's emergency number (e.g. USA, 911; UK 999). If no one in your group has a cellular phone, look for a nearby roadside emergency telephone or flag down a motorist to make the call. There is a good chance a passing motorist will have a cellular telephone.

7 Is a non-ambulance hospital visit required? Are there bone injuries or deformities? Is the rider unable to move an arm or leg easily? If so, he or she needs a trip to hospital. Even though it is possible that an ambulance is not required, an ambulance ensures faster treatment at hospital and may obviate the need for the individual to sit in a waiting room to register. If it is uncertain whether a trip is required, err on the side of caution.

8 Family contacts. Contact or make arrangements to contact family members or close friends of the injured rider if a hospital trip is needed.

Abrasions (road rash)

This, the most common of bicycling injuries, can be treated in different ways. The right way reduces healing time and scarring.

The severity of road rash is similar to that of burns:
1 First-degree: only the surface is reddened. This problem does not require active treatment.
2 Second-degree: the surface layer of the skin is broken, but a deep layer remains that will allow the skin to replace itself and heal without significant scarring.
3 Third-degree: the skin is entirely removed, perhaps with underlying layers of fat and other supporting tissue structures are exposed. Such damage may require skin grafting and is beyond the scope of this book. Seek immediate medical attention.

Treatment

The objective of treatment is to heal the tissues as rapidly and effectively as possible. Goals of therapy include preventing further damage to the skin and not allowing the depth of the rash to increase. However, some things can go wrong. The rash can heal with scarring. The rash can take longer to heal than needed, for example, because of infection. Or the rash can heal, but be more painful than necessary during the healing process.

There are two general methods of treatment for second-degree road rash. The first is the traditional 'let nature take its course', approach, which is also called the *open method*. This involves cleaning the wound with soap and water, hydrogen peroxide, an iodide or something similar, and then allowing the wound to dry out, form a scab and heal on its own.

This method has its drawbacks for all but the most superficial small road rashes. Just because abrasions have been cleaned once does not mean that they will not become infected. Bacteria thrive on damaged skin. Infection can deepen the depth of the abrasion, meaning that scarring and delayed healing are more likely. Scabs can crack and become painful. Scabbed areas do not receive oxygen well from the surrounding air, and so take much longer to heal.

The alternative is the *closed approach* – frequent cleansings and the application of topical antibiotics and dressings which keep the abrasion moist and closed to the air. The area is cleansed at least daily with wet compresses or bathing. Superficial debris is gently removed. An effort is made to remove soft-forming exudates (the beginnings of scabs) with gentle scrubbing. These exudates usually form between the third and fifth days after injury. Pink, healthy, new-forming skin is what you want to see. Second-degree road rash usually takes 2–3 weeks to heal.

Treatment supplies. Silver sulfadiazine (Silvadene), mupirocin (Bactroban) or Polysporin is applied. A petroleum jelly gauze (e.g. Adaptic) is placed over this. This is a non-stick mesh that allows the dressing to be removed without sticking. Padding in the form of gauze squares may be applied. Then, a conforming gauze roll is wrapped around the area and taped in place. Finally, a tube stretch gauze (e.g. Tubigauze) is applied over this to keep everything in place and tidy.

Alternatively, Tegaderm or Bioclusive alone may be stretched over the antibiotic.

The result is a dressing that allows maximum protection of the wound, minimum risk of infection, prevention of scabbing and its attendant cracking and pain, and healing as fast as possible.

Those who are allergic to sulphur drugs should avoid sulfadiazine. Mupirocin is slightly better at controlling skin infections, but is more expensive.

As the skin nears complete healing, it may be tempting to allow technique to become lax. Sun exposure may cause the skin to remain permanently darkened after healing. Be sure to keep abrasions covered until they are completely healed. Use adequate sunscreen with a sun protection factor of 15 or greater.

Collarbone fracture

The collarbone is the most common bone to break when a cyclist falls. It is usually the result of falling on an outstretched hand, causing indirect violence to the shoulder girdle.

Healing and treatment

Most bones heal or knit in about 6 weeks. The collarbone is no exception. As the collarbone heals it forms callus, or 'bone glue', where it was broken. This callus results in a thickened area. In many cases, the collarbone is stronger after it heals than it was before it was broken.

About 80% of the time the collarbone breaks between the middle and outer third. This type of fracture, where the bones are in good alignment, has an excellent prognosis. About 15% of the time the break is much closer to the acromioclavicular (AC) joint, in which case healing may be more difficult. Rarely, the break is near the sternum, or breast plate.

Most collarbone injuries will heal well without much medical or surgical intervention. A figure-of-eight bandage, which pulls the shoulders back, is sometimes prescribed for a couple of weeks. This may help keep the ends of the break in better alignment and reduce discomfort. Additionally, the arm is often placed in a sling. Most patients discard the sling and bandage after a week or two.

Occasionally the bones do not knit or form good callus, but heal loosely with only a fibrous connection. Surgery may be required in the unusual case where a collarbone injury does not heal on its own. Occasionally the break compresses a nerve, and surgery is required for decompression. Surgery may be advisable from the outset in some breaks close to the AC joint associated with significant ligament tearing.

Orthopaedic surgeons rarely perform surgery on broken collarbones in the USA. Their European counterparts are more likely to consider a surgical option in order to provide a faster return to racing.

Return to riding

For aligned collarbone breaks where normal healing is expected, in a very motivated athlete, training can resume almost immediately, usually in 48 h. Since jarring of the road is uncomfortable, training is performed on a stationary trainer. A specific workout plan is invaluable, as otherwise most riders waste their time. Raising the front of the trainer a little (6 cm) will allow the rider to ride in a more upright position with less weight on the shoulder and less pain.

Active shoulder exercises (see p. 90) may be begun when pain lessens, usually about 1 week after injury. Most riders with a fractured collarbone can ride on the road in about 2 weeks, especially on a hybrid or

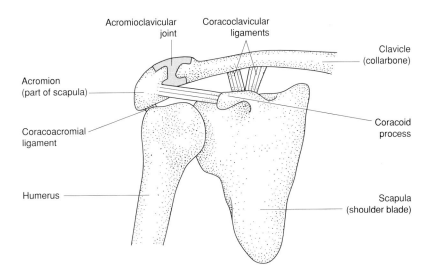

Fig. 6.9 Shoulder joint anatomy.
A shoulder separation is a stretching
or tearing of the shoulder ligaments.

mountain bike with fat tyres that absorb road shock.
Serious road riding and racing can resume, if all goes
well, in 4–6 weeks. Mountain bike racing may be
delayed another month.

The above are guidelines for motivated racers with
good breaks. Some riders have won national or world
championships a week after a collarbone fracture.
Others take several months to get back into the swing
of things.

Shoulder separation (AC sprain)

Shoulder separation or AC sprain are terms for a
stretching or tearing of the shoulder ligaments. The
collarbone meets the shoulder blade at the AC joint.
This is a point on the forward top part of the shoulder.
Injuries to this area by direct trauma in bicyclists are
common. Falls on the outward prominence of the
acromion tend to force it downward.

The clavicle is held to the shoulder blade at the AC
joint by a fibrous envelope or capsule. There are also
two coracoclavicular ligaments, which are fibrous
attachments between the clavicle and the coracoid
part of the shoulder blade (Fig. 6.9).

Shoulder separations are divided by severity and
X-ray appearance. X-rays may be taken with weights
on the affected arm to show any weakness of the
structures.

1 First-degree separation: the capsule is stretched but
not completely torn. There is local pain at the AC

joint, which worsens with abduction (raising outward) of the arm. X-rays do not show any movement at
the AC joint.

2 Second-degree separation: capsule disruption
is such that the X-ray shows some movement of the
acromion downward relative to the clavicle. This
displacement is less than the width of the clavicle.

3 Third-degree separation: the separation is as much
as or more than the width of the clavicle. The coracoclavicular ligaments have been torn. An operation
may be necessary.

Treatment

First- and second-degree separations are treated with a
sling. Range-of-motion exercises may begin when pain
allows, usually within a week of the injury. Stationary
trainer workouts may begin almost immediately. Road
riding and racing can commence as discomfort allows.
Third-degree separations may take as long as
6 weeks to heal on their own. Some orthopaedic
surgeons prefer operative treatment of third-degree
separations.

Shoulder dislocation

Anterior or posterior dislocations of the shoulder are
usually reduced in emergency rooms. Always check
neurovascular status before reduction. Although
reduction can take place in the field, either the

original injury or the reduction can cause a fracture. X-ray control before reduction properly identifies those fractures antecedent to reduction. A sling is often prescribed for discomfort. Although training on a stationary trainer may resume almost immediately, many physicians believe that keeping the arm in a sling for three weeks, together with physical therapy, helps prevent recurrent dislocation.

Shoulder injury exercises

Pendulum exercises

These exercises are performed with about 2.5 kg weight in the hands. Exercises can be done while standing and leaning over. Ideally, they are performed on a bench, facing downwards.
1 Move the arm forward and backward, allow the weight in the hands to help develop swing.
2 Do the same exercise, side to side.
3 Make circles in one direction, getting wider and wider; then go in the other direction.

Wall climbing

1 Face the wall with outstretched hands and with the fingertips just touching the wall. Walk the fingertips up the wall. Gradually and slowly walk towards the wall as the fingertips travel higher. Repeat 10 times.
2 Do the same thing facing sideways to the wall. Starting with the fingertips near the side, move slightly away from the wall to allow the fingers to creep up to the horizontal. As they rise above the horizontal, approach the wall again.

Ankle sprain

Ankle sprain is the stretching or tearing of ligament fibres that support the outside or the inside of the ankle. If the injury is to the lateral aspect of the ankle, if there is not much swelling or tenderness over the bones of the ankle, if gait is normal, and if there is no ecchymosis (blood bruising of the skin), self-treatment may be tried.

Ankle sprains are divided into three groups. Grade 1 sprains are the least severe, while grade 3 are the most severe.
1 Grade 1 sprains involve tearing of less than 20% of the ligament fibres. They have minimal swelling, and

weight bearing is with little or no pain. There is no ecchymosis.
2 Grade 2 sprains involve tearing of 20–70% of the ligament fibres. They have moderate swelling, and walking is difficult. Blood bruising of the skin is usually present.
3 Grade 3 sprains involve tearing of more than 70% of the ligament fibres. Swelling is moderate or severe. Walking is impossible. Blood bruising of the skin is present.

Causes

Most sprains result from an inward twisting motion of the foot and most of the time the lateral ankle is sprained. Occasionally it is the medial aspect that has the problem. The cause is not usually cycling-related *per se*. Sprains usually occur just as they occur in non-riders, for example, by stepping into a pothole or off a pavement.

Treatment

All sprains are treated initially with RICE – rest, ice, compression and elevation. All are treated with anti-inflammatory and pain medicines as needed. An X-ray is usually needed to make sure no fracture is present.

Grade 1 sprains may be treated with a weight-bearing brace or strapping for a couple of weeks. Ace wraps usually do not provide much support; a Coban bandage (3 m product, a self-adherent elastic wrap that functions like tape) or athletic strapping provides better support.

Grade 2 sprains are treated as for grade 1 sprains. Additional support may be needed for longer. An air-cast ankle brace or other support may be helpful. A weight-bearing shoe may be needed for a few weeks. Crutches are usually used. Flexion–extension exercises are begun after 48 h. Full ankle range-of-motion exercises are begun a couple of weeks after the injury.

Grade 3 sprains may need an air-cast or traditional cast for several weeks. Surgery may be required.

Cleats that allow too much float may aggravate ankle sprains.

Complications

All sprains are associated with frequent reinjury. Inadequate rest can delay healing and cause a relatively minor sprain to persist longer than it would otherwise. Persistent swelling following an ankle sprain is common. Occasionally the initial injury, combined with the repeated stress of riding, causes tendinitis. If, even with proper support, riding worsens pain, it is sensible not to ride until the injury is healed. Severe sprains may result in long-term ankle weakness and instability, requiring surgery.

Head injury and helmet use

Head injury is the most common cause of cycling-related death.

1 In the USA, about 1000 bicycling deaths each year are caused by head injuries.
2 About 80% of all cycling deaths result from head injuries.
3 Sixty to 70% of all serious bicycle injuries involve head trauma.
4 Fifty per cent of head-injury deaths occur in adults, 50% in children and adolescents.
5 Head-injury rate is reduced by as much as 85–95% by using a helmet.

Concussion is an injury to the brain, usually related to a blow to the head. Any concussion is potentially dangerous. The longer one is unconscious, or the longer the memory loss, the worse the concussion. Concussion can be serious even without losing consciousness, being cut or having a bump on the head. Concussion can result in permanent brain damage and death.

Athletes should be advised to seek medical attention if any of the following develop:

1 loss of consciousness;
2 convulsions;
3 memory loss;
4 confusion;
5 restlessness and irritability;
6 garbled speech;
7 vomiting more than once;
8 unusual sleepiness or decreasing alertness;
9 double vision;
10 pupils of different sizes;
11 trouble using arms or legs;
12 fever;
13 bleeding from the nose or ears;
14 headaches that do not ease up, especially headache not directly underneath the area struck.

To be effective, a helmet must be properly fitted. It needs to be the right size, worn covering the top of the forehead, and the straps must be snug. A number of helmet safety standards exist, including those of the American National Standards Institute (ANSI) and the Snell Memorial Foundation. Approved helmets carry a sticker.

Once crashed, helmets lose much of their effectiveness and should be replaced. Helmet materials deteriorate with age. Helmets should be replaced at least every 5 years.

As in other professional sports, whenever new safety equipment is introduced, there is often resistance to the adoption of such equipment. For example, when hockey helmets were first introduced, complaints were loud and strong. After a few years, or even a generation of athletes, such safety requirements tend to be not only adopted, but embraced by all.

Although a particular individual may desire the freedom to choose not to use safety equipment, in many countries it is the state that pays health-care costs. The state may impose safety requirements in sport, as it does in the use of seat belts in cars. Professional riders are seen as role models and have a responsibility to others as well as to themselves.

Heat is not an issue. Although wearing a helmet when resting is hotter, modern well-ventilated helmets have no significant effect on overheating while riding on hot days: some studies have even shown a cooling effect. Aerodynamics is improved compared with riding bare-headed. Weight is of trifling significance; helmets weigh about 0.25 kg. Nor is cost is an issue; the cost is a fraction of a single emergency room visit, and about the same as a routine doctor's office visit.

Internal medical problems

A number of internal medical problems are caused by cycling. Other problems, although not caused by cycling, are worsened by it. Still others require modification or consideration in treatment because of cycling activities. Internal medical problems associated with cycling are discussed below.

Muscle cramps

Cramps are involuntary muscle contractions or spasms, which are often sustained and painful. Muscle cramps can and do affect almost all riders.

Causes

There are many causes of cramps. It is difficult to be certain why cramps occur in any individual. Although many suggestions have been offered to help prevent cramps, there is probably as much folklore as science in most recommendations. Some of the more likely causes are:

1 fluid and electrolyte imbalance. This is probably more of a problem in the local muscle-cell area than a reflection of overall body electrolyte imbalance or dehydration. Some of the electrolytes implicated are magnesium, potassium and calcium;
2 temperature changes – either unacclimatized cold or hot weather;
3 low blood sugar;
4 unaccustomed sudden hard exertion or inadequate conditioning;
5 fatigue;
6 waste product accumulation, such as lactic acid;
7 lack of flexibility;
8 medical problems or diseases.

Prevention

1 Train specifically. If there are surges and jumps in races, train that way.
2 Eat a diet rich in carbohydrates, calcium, potassium and magnesium.
3 Eat during long rides.
4 Be adequately hydrated before and during rides and races.
5 Allow time for acclimatization.

Treatment

1 Stretch or massage the cramp. The rider may be able to do this while continuing to ride, or the cramp may force him or her to stop.
2 Apply hot or cold packs.

Headache

Some cyclists experience headache during or after rides because of tightness in the neck muscles. Time triallists often experience this problem, related to holding the head in a craned position. Mountain bikers may experience this problem because of

jarring. Treatment is described under neck pain, above.

Exertional headache may be a variant of migraine, caused by a spasm in a blood vessel, rather than arising from muscle contraction.

Anti-inflammatory medication, such as over-the-counter aspirin, ibuprofen or naproxen, may help either preventively or after the fact. Preventive treatment with a variety of other prescription medications is also available. Some of these medications worsen athletic performance.

Rhinorrhoea and nasal congestion

A runny or congested nose is very common in cyclists. The nose does run more when cycling. Sometimes this is related to allergy or irritants in the air. The eyes produce more tears when riding, and the tears flow down through the tear ducts into the nose, causing more secretions.

Some riders use over-the-counter decongestants, antihistamines, or a combination of both to relieve symptoms. The side-effects of these medicines are usually not worth the minimal relief they provide.

Respiratory infections

Aspirin or paracetamol (acetaminophen) helps ease aches and pains. Decongestants help stuffiness and runny noses. Be careful when using decongestants around the time of competition: they may be banned when present over a certain amount, or completely banned.

Fever is associated with considerably increased metabolic demands on the body. Go easy, or do not ride at all. Muscle aches are sometimes associated with rare, potentially more dangerous infections that may cause complications with the increased stress of training, for example, cardiomyopathy. If muscle aches are associated with infection, it is wise to rest.

If fever and muscle aches are present, but there are no symptoms above the neck – no sore throat and no nose symptoms – use caution. Exercise may significantly worsen some virus-caused conditions that fit this description.

When the colour of sputum or nasal discharge is yellow or green it often signifies a bacterial infection.

If this lasts more than a few days or is associated with fever, antibiotics may help.

Dyspnoea (not enough air)

The feeling that one cannot get enough air is a common medical problem. It occurs in cyclists whether in the presence or absence of disease.

Breathing is controlled by the nervous system in response to varied stimuli. Breathing rates can increase appropriately according to increased metabolic demands during exercise. Breathing can also increase without metabolic demands, for example, due to anxiety or fear.

Normally, individuals are not specifically aware of the act of breathing. With mild exertion, breathing rates may increase and a person may become more conscious of breathing, but discomfort is not felt. With heavy exertion, breathing may become unpleasant, but the individual is aware that this will be transitory, and that it is appropriate for the level of exercise.

Unlike the above, dyspnoea is the *abnormally uncomfortable awareness of breathing*. Dyspnoea relates to a change in the aerobic system's capabilities rather than to its absolute capacity (Fig. 6.10). A lack of air is perceived when there is a reduction in aerobic capacity from baseline.

For example, an athlete who has donated blood may still have twice the aerobic capacity of an untrained sedentary individual. The athlete whose aerobic capacity has been reduced by anaemia may feel dreadful on exertion and be acutely aware that there's 'not enough air'. The sedentary individual, whose aerobic capacity is much smaller but unchanged, may feel

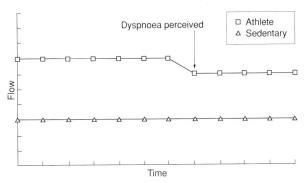

Fig. 6.10 Dyspnoea relates to a change in baseline, rather than absolute, lung function.

perfectly well and have no perception of any shortness of breath.

Causes

Dyspnoea is an aerobic system problem. The sensation of difficulty will be perceived to be in the lungs. The lungs may or may not be the problem.

In addition to the lungs, medical problems may be caused by the heart, by a hormonal problem such as thyroid disease, or by a metabolic factor affecting oxygen delivery to the muscle. Dyspnoea may also be related to environmental, non-medical problems.

Lung problems include obstruction to airflow due to asthma, bronchitis or emphysema. Blockage of the lung blood vessels (for example, due to a clot from a pulmonary embolus) commonly results in dyspnoea. Diseases of the chest or respiratory muscles also cause dyspnoea.

Heart disease, in many forms, is commonly associated with dyspnoea.

An example of a metabolic factor causing dyspnoea is anaemia. The lack of oxygen-carrying red blood cells results in an inadequate aerobic system. Shortness of breath with exertion may be the perceived symptom.

Environmental changes that cause dyspnoea include riding at higher altitude and unaccustomed riding in pollution.

Treatment

It is important to distinguish an abnormally uncomfortable awareness of breathing from the awareness of breathing all individuals experience with significant exertion. Treatment depends upon specific diagnosis.

Exercise-induced bronchospasm (EIB)

Many athletes complain of breathing problems during exercise. Some problems occur under any circumstances, while some are specific to exercise.

Greatly simplified, the common lung problems are:
1 asthma: spasm of the air tubes;
2 bronchitis: inflammation or infection of the air tubes;
3 emphysema: destruction of the air tubes, usually from smoking;
4 pneumonia: infection of the cells of the lung itself.

Normal breathlessness that occurs when cycling hard usually has more to do with the heart, blood vessels and muscle cells than it does with the lungs.

Many people suffer from asthma. The classic definition of asthma used to be 'reversible airways obstruction', implying that the spasm or obstruction of the air passages could be helped with medicine. The extent to which a lung problem could be reversed with medication reflected the degree of spasm. Modern thinking believes that, in addition to pure spasm, mucus-producing obstruction and inflammation are involved. It is now known that some effects of asthma on lung function are irreversible in patients with long-standing disease. Asthma shares the gene that predisposes to hayfever, allergic rhinitis and eczema.

Many people have asthma as a child and grow out of it. They are not aware that they have any lung problem. Others have mild symptoms related to their underlying tendency toward asthma. They may be aware that they wheeze only with a cold or the flu, or that their colds last longer than other people's.

Cold, exercise, dry air and pollution are other factors that bring on or worsen asthma. A cyclist often faces one or more of these exacerbants when riding. Many racers have problems with exercise-induced asthma, or EIB. These terms are commonly used interchangeably.

EIB affects perhaps as many as one-third of all racers and Olympic-endurance athletes.

Diagnosis

Many individuals are aware that wheezing is the hallmark symptom of asthma. Cough, however, is the most common feature of this problem. Chest tightness is a frequent symptom. With great enough exertion, most people will cough after stopping. Those with EIB will cough more frequently, for longer and after less exertion. Those with EIB may find that cold weather makes them cough more readily, even without anaerobic efforts.

Everyone becomes out-of-breath with significant exertion, so being out-of-breath is not of itself a reliable feature. *Caution*: heart disease may present similar symptoms. Sinusitis is sometimes misdiagnosed as a lung problem.

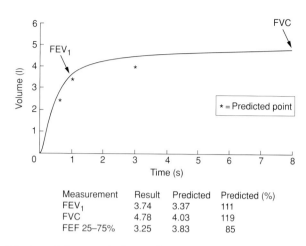

Measurement	Result	Predicted	Predicted (%)
FEV$_1$	3.74	3.37	111
FVC	4.78	4.03	119
FEF 25–75%	3.25	3.83	85

Fig. 6.11 Spirometry before medication.

A specific diagnosis can often be made with pulmonary function tests. This can be done with lung-measuring equipment. These devices measure change in lung function. They can also demonstrate how medicine helps to restore or improve breathing. Standard screening tests in many doctors' surgeries often do not uncover EIB. Cyclists may have symptoms with normal or near-normal screening lung function tests. Sometimes it may be necessary to test lung function during or after exercise or to give a trial of asthma medicine.

Figure 6.11 shows the results of forced exhalation spirometry of an elite female bicycle racer. The asterisks show the predicted lung function: her levels are better than normal.

The two most commonly used standard screening tests for lung function are: (i) the FEV$_1$, which represents the forced expiratory volume in 1 s (how much air one can breathe out in 1 s), and (ii) the FVC or forced vital capacity (the total amount of air one can breathe out). The FEV$_1$ and FVC shown in Fig. 6.11 are well above predicted: 111% and 119% of normal. Many practitioners would say this athlete's test is normal.

However, the most important screening test is the third measurement listed. It is the FEF 25–75%, or the forced expiratory flow between 25 and 75% of exhalation (the rate at which air is blown out in the middle part of the exhalation). As it is difficult to read it off the graph, it is computer-generated. This athlete's is 85%, which is not bad, but not good either.

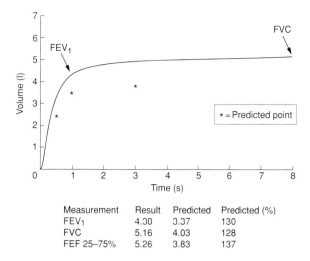

Measurement	Result	Predicted	Predicted (%)
FEV₁	4.30	3.37	130
FVC	5.16	4.03	128
FEF 25–75%	5.26	3.83	137

Fig. 6.12 Spirometry after medication.

Fig. 6.12 shows what happened when this cyclist was given an asthma medicine through a breathing machine and her lung function was retested 30 min later. The curve is much better. Her FEF 25–75% rose from 85% of normal to 137% of normal – more than a 50% increase. In her next race, which was an international stage race, this athlete was easily placed in the top 10, and felt better than she had done in months.

Treatment

1 A gradual warm-up helps prevent exercise-induced symptoms.
2 Nose-breathing, which helps increase the humidity of the air travelling to the lungs, may help.
3 Reduce exposure to common allergens and irritants. Common allergens include housemites found in housedust, flowers, certain weeds, trees and pets. Common irritants include pollution, smoke and home and workplace chemicals. Ammonia, for example, found in window and other cleaners, is a common home irritant.
4 If exposure to allergens and irritants is unavoidable, a facemask may help.
5 Remember that other illnesses such as colds and the flu worsen asthma.
6 Pre-exercise treatment with a variety of medications can help.

7 Regular medication can reduce symptoms in those in whom simple pre-exercise medication is insufficient. Inhaled medicines are usually improperly or inadequately used. One-on-one instruction with a health-care professional is almost always required.

Medical. A variety of inhalers are used to help prevent or treat EIB. The most common medicines belong to a class of medicines known as *adrenergic* agents. All medicines in this group can cause anxiety, tremor, nervousness or palpitations. These inhaler medicines are usually prescribed with a dose of two puffs, up to four times daily. If side-effects are a problem, a single puff may be taken.

The most frequently prescribed adrenergic medicine in the USA is albuterol (Ventolin and Proventil). Salmeterol (Serevent) is not marketed for EIB. It lasts longer than albuterol. Multiple overlapping doses have a potential for serious side-effects. Using only up to two puffs of salmeterol on days of competition, may be helpful, with relatively few side-effects.

Over-the-counter epinephrine (adrenaline) has more side-effects than the adrenergic inhalers mentioned above. Use a prescription inhaler instead.

Cromolyns (Intal, Tilade) are sometimes prescribed for EIB, but I have not found them to be as useful as the adrenergics.

Many patients walk out of the doctor's surgery with a prescription for an inhaled *steroid* (beclomethasone, truamcinolone, flunisolide). These medicines can be useful, but only if taken regularly, day after day. They do not work well for occasional use. They are, however, the drugs of choice for people who have persistent asthma (more than twice a week).

A common mistake is not receiving good instruction on the use of inhalers. In this author's experience, more than 75% of patients using inhalers do so incorrectly.

Some of the medicines used to treat EIB are banned by the International Olympic Committee. Some are legal for use only by physician registration. Remember that there is a difference between those medicines which are considered dangerous and banned medicines. If these medicines are indicated for treatment, registering their use is not bad: it helps to avoid the inference that they are being used for improved performance unrelated to a medical condition.

Although some athletes without EIB or asthma use these medicines for their perceived ergogenic benefit, it is doubtful whether they are useful except in the presence of disease.

Small hand-held peak airflow meters can be useful to help monitor asthma at rest and during rides. These devices cost about US$25 and fit into a jersey pocket. They can be used at home to help monitor baseline lung function. On rides they give information about how exercise is affecting the lungs, and how the lungs respond to medicine.

Gastrointestinal problems

This section is concerned with symptoms originating in the gastrointestinal (GI) tract related to exercise. Of course, many GI problems are not exercise-related. Some GI problems, such as diarrhoea caused by infection with *Giardia*, are not discussed here.

More than one-third of participants in exhausting endurance events experience one or more of the following problems:

1 GI shutdown: inability to take in fluids or solids;
2 heartburn or other acid problems;
3 diarrhoea;
4 cramps;
5 nausea or vomiting;
6 belching and gas;
7 bleeding – whether hidden or apparent.

During exercise how the body functions changes. It may take several hours after intense exercise for GI function to return to normal. The following alterations occur:

1 The normal emptying of the stomach is delayed.
2 The stomach contents back up into the oesophagus more easily than they do normally.
3 Stomach acid secretion decreases.
4 Peristalsis (the movement of the GI tract which propels food along) changes. Movement in the small intestine is slowed. Movement in the large intestine may increase.
5 Blood flow to the GI tract decreases: more blood goes to the working muscles in the legs. Blood flow may be reduced by up to 80%.
6 Blood flow occasionally decreases so much that the lack of blood causes bleeding of the bowel wall or stomach.
7 Nervous system activity changes.

8 Substances in the circulation, for example hormones and peptides, that affect the functioning of the GI tract change.
9 The absorption and secretion of substances in the lining of the GI tract change.

A number of factors make GI problems worse:

1 Level or intensity of exercise. As exercise intensity increases, the physiological changes described above increase. Whereas stomach emptying decreases by 80% or more with very high-intensity exercise, moderate exercise may decrease emptying by only 30%.
2 Dehydration. When the exerciser is already dehydrated, there is less blood volume for the body to spare from exercising muscle. Dehydration causes a vicious cycle: the more dehydrated one is, the more one needs fluids, yet the harder it is for the GI tract to accept them. The more dehydrated one is, the less well the stomach empties, and the less well the intestine absorbs fluids.
3 Heat and humidity. This is another vicious cycle. Heat and humidity force the body to shunt blood to the skin to aid in cooling. Heat and humidity increase sweat rates and worsen dehydration. Both these factors decrease the blood available to the gut. The need for fluids is increased, but the ability to handle them is worsened.
4 Concentrated liquids or solids. Ingesting fluids or solids that are hyperosmolar (that have a higher concentration than blood) worsens GI problems. The higher the concentration of fluids, the harder it is for the body to process them. Before concentrated fluids can be absorbed, their concentration must be neutralized to match the concentration of blood. This means that the lining walls of the gut must secrete fluids into the GI tract before the concentrated fluids consumed can be absorbed. Forcing the body to do this causes cramps, tightening of the gut and diarrhoea in many people. Modern carbohydrate energy bars and gels consumed without ample fluids commonly cause problems.
5 Fructose. Although fructose or fruit sugar has some important performance-enhancing properties, many find fruit juices or sodas containing it more difficult to tolerate than sports drinks containing glucose.
6 Fibre, fat and protein. All can contribute to GI distress in susceptible individuals. When compared with digestible carbohydrates, they slow the gut function and can cause digestive disorders.

7 Caffeine and alcohol. Caffeine and alcohol products cause many GI symptoms, even in people who do not exercise. They can certainly worsen symptoms in those who do.

8 Anxiety. Anxiety or stress commonly causes GI distress in both athletes and non-athletes. Some riders become so nervous before important rides or races that they cannot eat without distress for more than a day before their event.

Treatment

Pacing. Since increased exercise intensity worsens the functioning of the gut, it is prudent to pace oneself and not go out too hard.

Consider a century ride. Most riders can ride the first hour at 85% of maximum heart rate. But gut function would decrease substantially. Since most riders need to drink and eat even to get to the halfway point, it makes sense to ride closer to 75% of maximum for the first few hours.

Hydration. Remember that dehydration causes a vicious cycle. Keeping hydrated makes it easier to stay hydrated. If one starts out well-hydrated and keeps hydrated, it will be easier to sustain hydration. The stomach empties much faster with cool liquids than it does with warm or air-temperature ones. Some sugar and electrolytes in solution improve taste.

Avoid concentrated solutions: a 5% glucose solution might empty five times faster from the stomach than a 40% solution. Avoid certain food and drinks. There is great variety in what riders can successfully drink or eat. Some have success with certain drinks, while others cramp up with the same ones. Full-strength fruit juices, some full-strength energy drinks and fatty meals almost universally cause problems. Caffeine may help some riders perform, but may cause GI symptoms in many others. Experiment on training rides, not during big events.

Although it is popular to think that alcohol aids digestion, the reverse is often true.

Control of anxiety. This is perhaps easier said than done. Sometimes those new to racing just have to 'get their feet wet' and their pre-race anxiety will disappear. Others may need to give themselves a good talking to and get a grip on things. Some athletes benefit from a sports psychologist to help them channel their anxiety constructively.

Training. The gut probably does not become accustomed to intense exercise, but training improves its ability to function at a given work load. With training, more blood is available for the GI tract: a smaller percentage of the exerciser's maximal oxygen uptake is required at that given work load.

Men's health issues

Some bicycling problems are specific to men. Here are some issues of concern and suggestions for men's health.

Penile numbness

Men frequently find that their penis feels numb or has a pins-and-needles sensation during or after riding. The penis may feel asleep, swollen or 'not there'. Usually, just the shaft of the penis is the problem, but sometimes the numbness may extend to the scrotum and base of the genitals.

The problem is worse on long rides, and worse after time trialling or riding for prolonged periods bent over in the drops or aero bars.

The cause is pressure on the pudendal nerve. The nerve itself, or the small arteries which supply it, is compressed between the symphysis pubis pelvic bone and the bicycle seat. This causes a disturbance in the functioning of the nerve and the tissues it supplies.

The best treatment is prevention. The usual cause is riding bent over for too long. Take rests from this position. Stretch and remove the pressure from the genitals periodically by standing on the bike or otherwise changing position. Use a seat position that points the nose of the saddle down slightly more or lower the height of the seat. A padded or different saddle may be helpful – perhaps a differently shaped saddle with a different width. Padded bicycling shorts may help.

Occasional nerve disturbance in this area usually resolves rapidly when pressure is relieved. Normal sensation returns within minutes for most riders. Sometimes up to 24 h is required for the nerve to return to apparently normal function. Rarely, more than a day is required. The longer it takes for the nerve to return to normal, the more damage is done.

This problem has nothing to do with the ability of the body to produce testosterone, the male hormone. It is not related to ability to produce sperm. But a numb penis is sometimes an 'unfeeling' penis. Some may find problems obtaining an erection, although others who would otherwise achieve orgasm rapidly may find sexual activity is improved because of reduced sensation.

A numb penis should be avoided because of the possibility of permanent nerve damage.

Penile erection (priapism)

Priapism is erection of the penis not related to sexual arousal. The cause is the same as penile numbness, described above: pressure on the pudendal nerve. Treatment is as for penile numbness: reduce the pressure on the pudendal nerve.

Impotence

Impotence is the inability to obtain a satisfactory erection for sexual intercourse. It is not the same as infertility, which for a man means not having enough quality sperm. It is not unusual for riders to have occasional difficulties in sexual relations because of riding. Less commonly, bicycling causes permanent impotence.

The ability to achieve a satisfactory erection for sexual intercourse depends on several systems. The blood and the nerve supply to the genitals must be intact. The most important sexual organ – the brain – must also be in gear. Inability to maintain a satisfactory erection often involves a combination of these factors.

The nerve supply to the penis can be reduced by bicycle-seat pressure. Decreased sensation in the penis can contribute to reduced sexual performance. This problem is usually a temporary one, although accident and injury can cause prolonged problems. There are reports of prolonged nerve damage from long-lasting pressure.

Libido, or interest in sexual relations, depends on many factors, including testosterone. Studies have shown that athletes during their racing seasons have decreased levels of testosterone. In part this is related

to exertion, and in part to weight loss and low percentage of body fat. These factors, combined with the general exhaustion of training and racing, often result in decreased sexual activity.

Treatment. Avoid excessive compression of the genitals and nerve injury through proper bicycle position.

Consider modifying training or sexual schedule if the energy required to perform both activities is too great within a certain period of time.

Understand the physiological effects of significant training on overall energy levels and libido.

Urinating difficulties

Cycling-related pressure, leading to inflammation of the urethra or bladder tube, may cause frequent urination, dribbling, decreased urinary stream force, nighttime urination or burning on urination. Additionally, an infection may be a complication of this irritation.

Pressure on the pudendal nerve, causing penile numbness, can decrease sensation when urinating.

Riders aged over 40 may have difficulties related to the prostate. Hesitancy before urinating and dribbling after urinating are common problems with the prostate and, for many men, are a normal part of ageing. Since other medical conditions may also cause these problems, it is wise to check that the prostate is normal on general physical examination. It is controversial whether cycling can aggravate the prostate.

Pressure may be relieved by varying position, by using padded saddles, by using wider tyres with lower air pressure, by using suspension, or by using less stiff bicycles or recumbents.

Prostatitis

Prostatitis means inflammation of the prostate gland. The prostate is a walnut-sized organ between the rectum and urethra or bladder tube. True medical prostatitis is caused by an infection and treated with antibiotics. Since it is difficult for antibiotics to enter the prostate gland, treatment with antibiotics is usually given for many weeks, or recurrence is common.

An ache in the prostate area is not necessarily related to infection. Perhaps chronic swelling of the prostate is responsible. Past bacterial debris may cause a chronic immunological reaction. Or perhaps, as in many headaches and stomach aches, there is no disease, but the problem is related to stress or other unknown factors.

Although pressure on the prostate is said by some to result from bicycle riding, and may cause or aggravate typical prostate symptoms, many physicians doubt this. Most doctors doubt that infection of the prostate is related to cycling. Cancer of the prostate is not related to cycling.

Women's health issues

Some bicycling problems are specific to women. Here are some issues of concern and suggestions for women's health.

Nipple friction and pain

Riding sometimes results in irritation of the nipples. Clothing chafes at the skin, causing irritation. Once irritated, repeated rubbing only worsens the problem. Wet clothes are especially irritating.

A support bra may help. Wearing a light-weight undershirt under the jersey reduces skin rubbing and relieves irritation. Sometimes an adhesive plaster covering helps a particularly irritated nipple.

An emollient, such as petroleum jelly, may protect the skin and reduce irritation.

Wear layers, dress appropriately to the weather, and change out of wet clothes as soon as possible.

Bicycle seat discomfort

Whereas most men will find the same kinds of saddles comfortable, this is not the case for women. Most of us are aware that the shape of a woman's pelvis is different to that of a man's. In fact, there are three or four common shapes of female pelvis; some women have an android shape similar to men.

For this reason, the shape of a saddle that will provide the most comfort is an individual affair. Riders must often try differently shaped saddles to determine the type that matches their anatomy the best. Some saddles, marketed for women, are more likely to be comfortable.

Padding or no padding, gel-filled or not? The answer to these questions depends on the riding style.

Some thin seat covers allow an extra layer between the buttocks and the saddle, preventing chafing.

Sometimes problems of seat comfort are related to the general fit of a bicycle. Most bicycles are designed for men. Most bikes are sized with too long a top tube. This too-stretched-out position can make the seat uncomfortable near the pubic bone.

Seat position has traditionally been with the nose of the saddle pointed slightly up or level. Some women need the nose just slightly pointed down in order to be comfortable and avoid irritating the urethra (the tube that carries urine from the bladder).

The time-trialling position is the worst for most women. Improved flexibility may allow pelvis rotation, reducing pressure on the pubic area, while at the same time allowing a more bent-over aerodynamic position.

A numbing cream may occasionally be used in this area.

Sex before or after bicycling

For many women, riding places pressure on the vaginal and pubic areas. This pressure may result in local inflammation or irritation, including swelling and chafing. Since sexual activity often also places pressure on these areas and may cause similar soreness due to inflammation, some women have discomfort riding after sexual activities, and some women have difficulty with sexual activities soon after riding.

Placing more pressure on the buttocks and away from the pubic areas may be helpful. Spend more time riding on the tops than in the drops. Make sure bike fit is correct – not too stretched out, and the nose of the saddle not too high. A different saddle may help.

Vulvar swelling

Women who spend a lot of time on the saddle occasionally develop swelling of the external genital area, the vulva, usually on one side. Pain is not normally a problem. The cause of the condition is not precisely known. This problem is not considered dangerous.

Yeast infections

Vaginal yeast infections are caused by an overgrowth of *Candida* yeast, which is normally found in small quantities in the vagina. Factors contributing to this overgrowth include use of oral antibiotics and increased warmth and moisture.

Reduce the warmth and moisture in this area. Regular douching is not healthy for the vagina, although an occasional vinegar douche is not harmful. Over-the-counter or prescription vaginal antiyeast cream may be helpful.

Not all vaginal infections are caused by yeast. If one is unsure or the problem does not clear up with self-treatment, check on the cause.

Pregnancy

There is no good scientific proof that riding while pregnant is either good or bad. Pregnancy increases the physiological demands on the body. It makes temperature regulation more difficult, and excessive heat may be harmful to the developing fetus. It reduces the amount of glycogen and energy available for cycling. As the abdomen becomes larger, the centre of gravity rises, and balance is more difficult. Avoid situations that put one at risk for falling.

Assuming that the rider has not experienced problems with past pregnancies or the current one, she can ride normally for the first 6 months of the pregnancy, as long as exertions are limited to 80% of maximum heart rate and overheating is avoided. After 6 months of pregnancy, limit prolonged exertions to 70% of maximum heart rate.

Bladder infections

Most women know the feeling of burning and frequent urination that comes from a bladder infection. Such infections are usually caused by *Escherichia coli*, a bacterium commonly found in stool. It is a short distance from the anus to the urethra, the bladder-emptying tube. In women the urethra is very short, and once colonized by bacteria, a bladder infection develops easily. Wiping in the wrong direction, certain sexual practices and bicycle riding may all allow these bacteria easier access to the urethra and the bladder.

There are a number of ways to prevent bladder infections:

1 Avoid dehydration. Concentrated urine stings and causes similar symptoms. Drinking frequently results in frequent urination; this may help wash out bacteria, allowing the body to reduce the numbers of bacteria on its own.

2 Do not put off urinating. Procrastination may allow the bladder to swell, reducing the amount of blood that nourishes it, and making it more susceptible to infection.

3 Urinate after sexual activity and riding.

4 Avoid pressure on the pubic area by correct seat position.

5 An acid urine prevents bacterial growth. One way to keep the urine healthy and acidic is to take 1 g vitamin C (ascorbic acid) daily. Alternatively, 1 g of aspirin (three regular-strength tablets) will also help acidify the urine.

Pressure or chafing irritation of the end of the urethra from a bicycle seat may cause the same symptoms without a true bacterial infection. Or, the irritation may weaken the surface of the urethra, allowing bacteria to grow, and resulting in an infection.

Prescription antibiotics are effective in the treatment of bladder infections. Prompt cure of this problem is expected in almost all patients.

Tampons

Do not leave the string of a tampon outside the vagina when riding. It is often rubbed by the saddle, and the chafing may cause irritation. If flow is so heavy that one tampon is insufficient, try two tampons, side-by-side at the same time. This can be much more comfortable than using a tampon and a pad.

Excessive leanness

There is no question that those with extra weight would do well to shed a bit. Excessive fat is just extra poundage one has to lug up hills, accelerate to speed with jumps and otherwise metabolically support.

However, excessive leanness, especially in women, is associated with eating disorders, menstrual irregularities or the loss of menstruation, and osteoporosis.

Excessive leanness may also hamper the immune system and lower resistance, making one more susceptible to colds, the flu and other infections. Excessive leanness may inhibit recovery and foster greater fatigue.

Athlete triad

The female athlete 'too-thin' triad consists of disordered eating, amenorrhoea (loss of periods) and osteoporosis. Some studies have shown that over one-half of athletic women have components of this triad. Old bones in young athletes are a serious problem. More information is found in the section on osteoporosis, below.

Body fat goals

A reasonable ideal level of body fat for a top-level female racer is 10–15%; for a top-level male racer, it is 5–10%. Some females do reduce to 6–8%, and some males reduce to 3–4%. But such leanness is not for everyone.

If you are always tired, cranky and overstressed, consider letting weight rise a few pounds and see if your mood improves. Those women who are thin enough to have stopped their periods should consider supplementing their diets with extra calcium and hormone treatment – most easily available in the form of birth-control pills – to help prevent osteoporosis.

Leanness can improve athletic performance, but it is not necessarily healthy.

Osteoporosis

Osteoporosis (low bone density, or thinning of the bones) is a common health problem in women, especially after the menopause, and an occasional problem in men. Weakened bones are more likely to break. Endurance and high-intensity cyclists often have irregular menstrual periods and altered hormonal status, which places them at risk for osteoporosis and future bone fractures.

Women often know their weight, blood pressure, cholesterol level and percentage body fat. They often do not know the status of their bone health.

There are a number of risk factors:

1 reduced cumulative oestrogen exposure: delayed onset of menstruation, early menopause, absent or irregular periods;

2 family history of osteoporosis or a history of low bone density;

3 nutrition, including low calcium and vitamin D intake, eating disorders and low calorie intake;

4 high level of physical activity;

5 thin and small body;

6 white or Asian race;

7 stress or low-trauma fractures;

8 medications, including thyroid hormone replacement, corticosteroids and phenytoin;

9 smoking;

10 high alcohol intake;

11 high caffeine intake;

12 diseases, including intestinal malabsorption.

A woman of any age who has prolonged oestrogen deficiency, resulting in irregular or absent periods, or other risk factors should be considered for a bone density measurement to evaluate bone health. Bone density can be measured at various sites and by various technologies. If only one measurement is made, the site usually examined is the lumbar spine in women younger than 65 and the femoral neck in women aged 65 and older.

Prevention and treatment

1 Nutrition: calcium intake should be 1500 mg daily. Calcium can be obtained from the diet or from pill supplements. Dairy products, dried beans, sardines and broccoli are high in calcium. Vitamin D helps calcium absorption.

2 Improve oestrogen levels: before the menopause, reduced exercise duration or intensity, increased caloric intake or oestrogen replacement with oral contraceptives may help. After the menopause, oestrogen replacement therapy has been shown to prevent osteoporosis.

3 Weight-bearing exercise: weight lifting and walking are associated with improvement. Cycling is not weight bearing. Long-distance cycling is associated with a worsening of osteoporosis.

4 Stop smoking.

5 Medical prescription therapy: new therapies, in addition to oestrogen, include bisphosphonates and calcitonin.

Oestrogens and birth control pills

Oestrogens are female hormones. The supraphysiological amounts in birth-control pills suppress ovulation. Replacement oestrogens are frequently prescribed for postmenopausal women when their naturally occurring levels wane.

There are pros and cons in the use of oestrogens. A few early studies showed that oestrogens may slightly decrease aerobic metabolism and promote fluid retention, thereby adversely affecting performance. When given to postmenopausal women without progesterone, oestrogens slightly increase the risk of uterine cancer. This risk is minimized by using progesterone as well. Oestrogens significantly reduce osteoporosis and cardiovascular disease. A few studies suggest that they may reduce the risk of Alzheimer's disease.

Birth-control pills usually reduce menstrual bleeding and are associated with reduced anaemia. They often help menstrual irregularities and cramps, allowing athletes to train more consistently and predictably.

Anaemia

Anaemia is a deficiency of the red blood cells. Transport of oxygen and carbon dioxide and buffering of acids are vital functions which must be operating optimally for an athlete to have best performance. If an athlete is anaemic, this will be a problem.

The main function of the red blood cell is to transport haemoglobin. Haemoglobin is the blood protein that carries oxygen from the lungs to the tissues. Red blood cells also contain the enzyme carbonic anhydrase, which speeds up the reaction between carbon dioxide and water. This reaction helps the blood to transport carbon dioxide from the tissues to the lungs.

Haemoglobin is also an excellent acid–base buffer. Buffering is necessary to help neutralize exercise-produced lactic acid. Red blood cells are responsible for about 70% of the buffering power of the blood.

Anaemia is usually determined by analysing blood to determine how much haemoglobin it contains or the percentage of red blood cells found (Table 6.2).

Red blood cells are produced in the bone marrow. Insufficient red blood cells mean that not enough oxygen can be transported. Too many red blood cells increase the thickness of the blood and slow blood flow. The numbers of red blood cells produced are regulated by the amount of oxygen reaching the tissues. Lack of oxygen in the tissues is sensed by the kidneys, which produce natural erythropoietin. Erythropoietin stimulates the bone marrow to produce more red blood cells.

Table 6.2 Blood tests in anaemia and their normal values.

	Male	Female
Hb	13–18 g · dl⁻¹	11.5–16.0 g · dl⁻¹
Hct	39–54%	35–48%
Serum iron	40–170 µg · ml⁻¹	40–170 µg · ml⁻¹
Ferritin	20–450 ng · ml⁻¹	10–350 ng · ml⁻¹

Haemoglobin (Hb): the quantity of haemoglobin in a sample of blood, measured in grams per decilitre.
Haematocrit (Hct): the percentage of blood made up of red blood cells.
Serum iron: the amount of iron in the blood, measured in micrograms per millilitre.
Ferritin: a form of storage iron, measured in nanograms per millilitre.

Some of the factors that may deprive the tissues of oxygen include blood loss due to bleeding, destruction of the bone marrow by radiation, high altitude, diseases that slow the circulation of blood to the tissues and exercise. All these conditions result in increased production of red blood cells by normal bone marrow.

Androgens, or male hormones, are found in both men and women. *Testosterone* is the most important male hormone. Red blood cell production is increased in response to androgens. The much higher levels of androgens found in men contribute to the increased production of red blood cells in postpubertal males. This is one reason why men have haemoglobin levels about 10% greater than women.

Erythropoietin is taken by some athletes in a synthetic form to enhance performance. It is a banned substance. Although it may improve performance, it also increases the thickness of blood and is associated with an increased risk of stroke, heart attack and death. These risks are great, making it very dangerous.

Iron is important in the formation of haemoglobin. About 65% of the iron in the body is in the form of haemoglobin. Storage iron, or ferritin, makes up about 25% of iron in the body. Myoglobin, an iron-containing compound found in muscles, makes up about 4% of iron in the body.

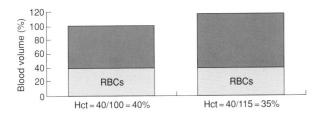

Fig. 6.13 Physiological anaemia. The total number of red blood cells (RBCs) is unchanged but the haematocrit is reduced.

The average amount of iron in the body is about 4 g. Males lose about 0.6 mg daily in the stool. Females lose about 2 mg daily. The increased average daily loss in females is as a result of the loss of blood during menstruation.

Folic acid and vitamin B₁₂ are needed to produce red blood cells. A deficiency of either results in a reduced number of red blood cells, and red blood cells that are larger than normal.

Normal red blood cells have an average life of 120 days. Abnormalities in the size or shape of red blood cells are sensed by the spleen, which acts as a filter, removing old or deformed red blood cells from the circulation.

If red blood cells are not properly formed, they do not last as long as 120 days. Even if an average number of red blood cells are produced, abnormalities in the formation of red blood cells may also lead to anaemia.

Causes

Sport anaemia. This is not related to iron deficiency. Many athletes have an increased volume of blood. The total number of red blood cells present in the circulation may be normal or mildly increased, but because the relative volume of blood in the circulation is increased, the concentration of red blood cells is reduced. The oxygen-carrying capacity of the circulation is unchanged or increased. This is athletic physiological anaemia and does not represent disease (Fig. 6.13).

Suppose the haematocrit – the percentage of red blood cells – is 40%. If the number of blood cells remains the same, and the volume of the circulation increases by 15%, the percentage of red blood cells will fall to 35%.

In some elite athletes, the high volume and intensity of exercise reduce testosterone production. Decreased testosterone production may contribute to sport anaemia.

Blood-loss anaemia. Blood loss from injury or blood donation may cause a rider to be anaemic until the body can replace red blood cells. It may take 4–6 weeks to replace a pint of blood, if all the building blocks for blood are present.

Iron-deficiency anaemia. This is the most common medical cause of anaemia. Women with heavy periods are most susceptible to this type of anaemia. Blood donors are also at risk of using up their iron stores.

When anaemia is discovered, the amount of iron or ferritin in the blood can be measured. If these are low, iron deficiency is diagnosed.

This type of anaemia is corrected by obtaining extra iron from iron supplements. Ferrous sulphate, which is easily purchased at the grocery store or pharmacy, is the supplement most often used.

Iron deficiency usually results from loss of iron in blood which is greater than that replaced by diet. It is important to look for a cause of bleeding if one is not readily apparent. Merely replacing the lost iron will not solve the problem.

Folic acid or vitamin B₁₂ deficiency. Deficiency of either one of these vitamins causes anaemia. Folic acid deficiency is one of the most common vitamin deficiencies in athletes.

Hormone-related anaemia. Decreased testosterone production, occurring in men as they age, decreased thyroid function, kidney failure, liver problems and alcoholism are all associated with anaemia.

Bone-marrow problems. Bone-marrow disease related to radiation exposure, industrial chemicals, drugs or cancer can cause anaemia.

Increased destruction of red blood cells. Sickle-cell anaemia, thalassaemia and other abnormalities of haemoglobin formation, immune problems and a deficiency of the enzyme glucose-6-phosphate dehydrogenase all result in the increased destruction of red blood cells.

Anaemia is a serious barrier to athletic performance. Although iron deficiency is the most common cause, it must not be assumed that anaemia is caused by iron deficiency. Proper medical diagnosis and the determination of any underlying causes will help correct the problem and optimize performance.

High blood pressure

High blood pressure, or hypertension, is a common medical condition. It is unusual to have symptoms in high blood pressure. Most of the time there is no known cause.

It is normal for blood pressure to vary from doctor visit to doctor visit. In fact, it is normal for blood pressure to vary from minute to minute. What counts in the diagnosis of hypertension is if blood pressure remains consistently high.

Treatment

Hypertension may initially be treated with salt restriction, alcohol restriction, weight reduction and exercise. If these measures are not successful, there are many effective medicines to treat this problem. At least three classes of high-blood-pressure medicines – diuretics, beta-blockers and calcium-channel blockers – may interfere with athletic performance.

Diuretics, or water pills, are good medicines for high blood pressure. They are often the first medicines selected in the treatment of hypertension. They are cheap, effective and usually need to be taken only once a day. Unfortunately, diuretics make one more susceptible to dehydration and interfere with performance.

Beta-blockers are also a common class of medicines used in the treatment of high blood pressure. They too are effective, have few side-effects and are relatively inexpensive. Many need to be taken only once a day. Beta-blockers are also used to treat heart disease, to prevent migraine, and to reduce stage fright or performance anxiety. They limit the work load that the heart can accomplish. This can be an extremely important benefit in heart disease. Beta-blockers are a poor choice for the performance athlete. If used effectively for medical disease, the heart rate may not be able to be raised to anaerobic threshold levels or beyond.

Calcium-channel blockers may limit the heart rate or reduce the force of contraction of the heart. This is especially true of verapamil (Calan, Isoptin). This may be a problem for some athletes.

Angiotensin-converting enzyme or ACE inhibitors are first-line antihypertension medications that are least likely to interfere with athletic performance. Unfortunately, they are relatively expensive.

Diabetes

Diabetes is an endocrine (hormonal) problem in which either a lack of insulin or a lack of responsiveness to insulin results in a number of metabolic problems. Insulin is produced in the pancreas. Most adults with diabetes are overweight. Weight reduction with diet modification and exercise will control or eliminate the signs and symptoms of diabetes in most of these individuals.

Diabetics may take medicine by mouth to increase the body's responsiveness to the insulin it already produces, or may take insulin by injection to replace what is not made. Those who must take insulin in order to prevent relatively immediate, serious complications are classified as having *insulin-dependent diabetes*. Much of the discussion below concerns insulin-dependent diabetes. This information is not a substitute for individualized, professional diabetic care.

The two most common types of insulin used are neutral protamine Hagedorn (NPH) (intermediate-acting) and regular (short-acting) (Table 6.3). Key to understanding their use is understanding the pharmokinetics or time actions of these products. Most diabetics take a combination dose of NPH and regular insulin in the morning and at night. Typically,

Table 6.3 Two common insulin preparations and their pharmokinetics.

	NPH	Regular
Onset	1–2 h	15–30 min
Peak action	8 (4–12) h	2–5 h
Duration of action	18–24 h	6–8 h

NPH, neutral protamine Hagedorn.

about 70% of the total daily dose is taken in the morning, and about 70% of each dose is NPH. A typical insulin-dependent diabetic might take 25/10 (25 units of NPH, and 10 of regular) in the morning and 10/5 in the evening.

Carbohydrates are absorbed from the GI tract into the blood stream. The actions of insulin result in blood sugar (glucose) being stored in tissues. Insulin allows blood-stream sugar to be stored in the liver, muscle and other areas as glycogen, or to be transported to adipose tissue and be stored as fat.

The immediate problem for diabetics is high glucose levels in the blood. Without insulin, glucose stays in the blood stream, and glycogen in muscle, liver and other tissues is not made. Fat is overused as a source of energy, and ketones, which are acidic byproducts of fat metabolism, accumulate in the blood.

Balancing the role of insulin in lowering blood sugar, two other hormones – glucagon and adrenaline – raise blood sugar levels. Glucagon is also produced in the pancreas, and most insulin-dependent diabetics have a problem regulating this hormone. Adrenaline is produced by the adrenal glands. Insulin-dependent diabetics do produce this hormone, but adrenaline alone is often not sufficient to prevent low blood sugar.

Exercise problems

Diabetics face a number of problems with exercise. Exercise can result in blood sugar levels that are too low or too high. Exercising muscles use glucose for energy. The demand for glucose during exercise in non-diabetics is met, in part, by decreased levels of insulin, which promote liver glucose production and glucose release into the blood stream for use by working muscles. Since exercise lowers blood sugar levels, insulin-dependent athletes who do not take this into account by reducing the amount of injected insulin risk low blood sugar or hypoglycaemia. The symptoms include sweating, nervousness, dizziness, tremor, hunger, weakness, palpitations and headaches.

If exercise is begun with already high blood sugar (and low insulin) levels, exercise may worsen the situation and create even greater hyperglycaemia. Glucagon levels rise and increase liver glucose pro-

duction. Low insulin levels result in less glucose and more fat-energy use by working muscles. Since high-intensity exercise is dependent upon glucose metabolism, performance will be impaired.

Since storage carbohydrate or glycogen is crucial for high-level performance, and since the making of glycogen is impaired in diabetics, high-level performance may be compromised even when blood sugar levels are optimum during exercise.

The kidneys help to normalize blood-sugar levels by flushing out excess sugar. Their increased action in imperfectly controlled diabetics makes dehydration more likely.

Temperature regulation in diabetes is often impaired. Exercise in hot and humid conditions imposes additional demands and risks.

Exercise benefits

1 Improved control of blood sugar and increased sensitivity of muscles to insulin: this may last several days.
2 Reduced cardiovascular risks.
3 Weight loss.
4 Psychological: stress reduction and a sense of well-being.

Exercise risks

1 Harder control with low and high blood sugars.
2 Orthopaedic or foot injury.
3 Accelerated degenerative joint disease.
4 Risks of worsening high blood pressure.
5 Possible increased microvascular (including kidney and eye) complications.

Exercise guidelines

1 Avoid beginning exercise with blood sugar levels below 70 mg · dl^{-1}.
2 Avoid beginning exercise with blood sugar levels above 300 mg · dl^{-1} if ketones are present.
3 Avoid dehydration. Drink before, during and after exercise.
4 Ingest about 25 g (420 J or 100 cal) of carbohydrate for every 30 min of intense exercise.
5 Have a recovery snack of carbohydrate after exercise.

6 Decrease the insulin dose. Omit a short-acting dose before exercise. Decrease the dose of intermediate-acting insulin on the day of exercise. Infusion/pump: eliminate meal-time bolus before and after exercise.

7 Be especially cautious about exercising at the peak of insulin action if no adjustment in the insulin dose has been made.

8 Avoid thigh injections of insulin for at least 2 h before exercise.

Moderately hard 1 h rides. After-breakfast morning or commute rides can be relatively easily managed by omitting the morning insulin dose of regular insulin, and by eating a little extra before, during and after the ride. Afternoon rides are managed by reducing the morning NPH insulin dose. Typically, only one-half of the NPH dose is taken.

Prolonged rides. The absolute amount of stored liver glycogen cannot meet glucose demands for prolonged high-level performance, even in non-diabetics. There is more reliance on fat metabolism. Just as non-insulin-dependent diabetics need to consume calories before, during and after rides, so insulin-dependent diabetics need to try and optimize carbohydrate use for prolonged rides, not only to manage their diabetes, but also to increase performance.

Travel and climate problems

The body's acclimatization to a new geographic environment may represent a trivial adaptation. Occasionally, it can be extreme and life-threatening. Common travel and climate effects include time-zone adaptation, cold, heat and humidity and altitude.

In general, increase fluid and complex carbohydrate consumption. Reduce fat and proteins and avoid caffeine, alcohol and simple carbohydrates.

Time-zone change

It is usually easier travelling from west to east than from east to west. Crossing one or two time zones usually presents no significant problem. Three or four time zones present challenges, and crossing five or more time zones requires at least several days for adaptation.

One can partially preadapt by rising an hour or two earlier or later, and retiring an hour or two earlier or later, depending on whether one is travelling east or west.

Some riders keep their watches on home time. This is a mistake. It is important to set the watch to the new time zone on arrival. It helps to adapt psychologically to the new time, and prevents missing race start times.

Travel tends to make most people tried. Travel is hard work. Do not worry if a day or two of training is missed.

If one is to cross many time zones, try and stay up and go to bed at the right time in the new time zone. A sleeping pill may help readjust the internal clock when used for a day or two. It often takes 1 day for each time zone crossed to feel and perform at potential.

Cold

Muscles have an optimal operating temperature. Warm-up helps them reach this level. Cold-weather riding makes it difficult for muscles to function well.

Tights and other protective gear can help performance significantly. Most riders perform better with tights when the temperature drops below 18°C on cloudy days or 15°C on sunny days. A thin layer protecting against wind chill is often all that is needed. Wind-shell jackets, long-fingered gloves and head-bands are also useful as the temperature falls.

Since cold weather decreases muscle performance and work, it also results in a lower Vo_{2max} and heart rate. Other things being equal, cold air is denser air: aerodynamics are worse and result in slower speeds. A 12°C drop in air temperature results in about a 1 min increase in time-trial time per hour.

Heat

This section covers how heat affects cycling performance, causing heat illness, and how the effects of heat can be minimized. This is especially important in races of more than a couple of hours.

When it is hot we sweat. Blood flow to the skin helps to shunt heat from the body's core. But it is not really sweating that cools, so much as evaporation of the sweat. That's why tail-wind climbs are so difficult in hot and humid conditions. A good head wind will slow you down but help keep you cool.

Heat affects performance in a number of ways:

1 Heat normally decreases the time necessary for warm-up.

2 Heat and humidity increase sweating, which increases dehydration and decreases performance.

3 Heat increases the heart rate for a given work load, increases maximum heart rate and decreases endurance cycling performance.

4 Heat increases the demands placed on the body: metabolism is speeded up and blood is shunted to the skin, so that less energy is available for working muscles.

5 Although hot air is lighter, heat is usually associated with high-pressure weather systems. Time-trial times may be lowered because of increased air density.

6 Drugs and alcohol may worsen heat tolerance. Beta-blockers and diuretics (used for high blood pressure), antihistamines and sedatives are known to worsen heat tolerance.

In conditions of high heat and humidity, a maximum of up to $5 \text{ l} \cdot \text{h}^{-1}$ may be lost at high exertion levels. That represents a water bottle every 7–8 min. Most of the time, fluid loss is less than the maximum; normally a bottle every 15–20 min is sufficient. Fluid loss can be estimated by weighing before and after rides. A 0.5 l water bottle weighs 0.5 kg.

Fluid loss sets up a vicious cycle. When hot, you need to sweat more. But when dehydrated, the sweat rate is reduced. With reduced sweat rate, you cannot lessen body heat. The sensation of thirst means dehydration is already present. Drink before you become thirsty.

The major electrolyte lost in sweat is sodium: about 2.5 g (one-half teaspoon) of salt may be lost with each litre of sweat. Most daily diets contain enough sodium to replace the losses in 5 l of sweat. Potassium, magnesium and chloride are also lost, but are not usually a problem.

On hot and humid days, consuming up to 2.5 g (one-half teaspoon) of salt per litre of fluid replaced helps stimulate thirst and replenish lost sodium. Plain salt in plain water tastes vile. Commercial flavoured electrolyte replacement drinks taste better. The easiest, safest and most palatable way of anticipating or replacing lost sodium is by eating salty foods. As always with new nutrition, experiment before racing.

Heat illnesses

There are four major heat-related medical problems. Elements of more than one problem may be present at the same time, as they are a continuum:

1 Heat cramps: it is thought that an imbalance in the body's fluids and electrolytes contributes to this problem. Acclimatization, fluids and salt may help.

2 Heat exhaustion: symptoms are weak, rapid pulse, low blood pressure, headache, dizziness and weakness. Sweating may be reduced but the body temperature is not elevated to dangerous levels. Stop exercising and move to a cooler environment. Use water sponging and push fluids.

3 Exertional heat injury: symptoms are goose flesh, sensation of chilling, throbbing headache, weakness, perhaps dry skin, nausea, vomiting, unsteady gait, incoherent speech and loss of consciousness. Stop exercising and move to a cooler environment. Use cool water or ice sponging, showers or baths. Fans may be useful and push fluids.

4 Heat stroke: symptoms are mental confusion, convulsions, loss of consciousness and increased body temperature. Sweating may stop, and the skin may be dry and hot. Untreated, it may progress to death. Emergency treatment and aggressive lowering of the body temperature are required. Stop exercising and move to an air-conditioned environment. Use cool showers or ice baths, fans and chilled intravenous fluids.

Measuring heat

Just like cold and the wind-chill index, there are measures of the effect of heat humidity and radiant heat. Whereas wind chill makes temperatures seem colder to the body, humidity, which slows evaporation, makes temperatures seem hotter.

Heat-stress index. The heat-stress index (Table 6.4) takes into consideration the effect of humidity.

Wet-bulb thermometry. Evaporation will lower the temperature of a thermometer whose mercury bulb is covered with a wet wick – a wet-bulb thermometer. It is also possible to make training recommendations solely on the basis of the wet-bulb reading (Table 6.5).

Table 6.4 The heat-stress index.

Humid-ity (%)	Air temperature (°C)										
	21	24	27	29	32	35	38	41	43	46	49
0	18	21	23	26	28	31	33	35	37	39	42
10	18	21	24	27	29	32	35	38	41	44	47
20	19	22	25	28	31	34	37	41	44	49	54
30	19	23	26	29	32	36	40	45	51	57	64
40	20	23	26	30	34	38	62	51	58	66	
50	21	24	27	31	36	42	49	57	66		
60	21	24	28	32	38	46	56	65			
70	21	25	29	34	41	51	62				
80	22	26	30	36	45	58					
90	22	26	31	39	50						
100	22	27	33	42							

Heat-stress index	Possible effect
32–41	Heat cramps
41–54	Heat cramps or heat exhaustion likely
	Exertional heat injury or heat stroke possible
55+	Heat stroke a definite risk

The intersection of air temperature and humidity is the body's perceived level of heat stress.

Acclimatization

The body adapts to hot and humid environments. Adaptation takes 1–2 weeks. Age and gender are not significant factors, but adaptation is harder for the obese. Restricting fluids in training does not improve acclimatization. The first workouts in the heat and humidity should be light. Even after several days of acclimatization, workouts should not be performed at maximum intensity.

If planning to travel to a hot and humid environment, acclimatization may be helped by wearing additional clothing and taking saunas, steam baths and hot tubs whilst still at home.

Acclimatization improves the blood flow to the skin and lowers the threshold for the start of sweating. It also increases sweat output and lowers the salt concentration of sweat.

Table 6.5 Wet-bulb thermometry.

Wet-bulb reading (°C)	Recommendations
15	None
16–18	Warn of possible heat stress
19–21	Insist on fluid consumption
22–24	Rest periods and water breaks mandatory every 20–30 min
	Limit intense activity
25–26	Modify or stop activity
27	Cancel workout

There are a number of ways to help cope with heat and humidity:

1 Hydrate well before, during and after riding.
2 Increase intake of fluids and salt.
3 Wear light-coloured clothing.
4 Wear less clothing where clothing limits evaporation.
5 Drink cool fluids with calories and salt.
6 Sponge, spray or pour water (preferably chilled) over the helmet, clothes or body.
7 Use sunscreen, but avoid waterproof non-breathing types.
8 Trim long hair. Shave beards.
9 Wear a well-ventilated helmet.
10 Aspirin may help headache and possibly reduce body temperature.
11 Obtain physician consultation: consider reducing the use of some medicines, especially those for high blood pressure.

Performance (Figs 6.14 and 6.15)

Adaptations allow improved physical performance, but this improved performance is never as good in tropical conditions as it is in moderate climates. Muscles have an optimal operating temperature. Exercise generates body heat. Hot bodies do not perform well. The body cools itself through sweating. When the body is hot, more blood flows to the skin to aid in sweating, and less is available for muscles. This decreases muscle performance and work. Dehydration is more likely, and this also decreases performance.

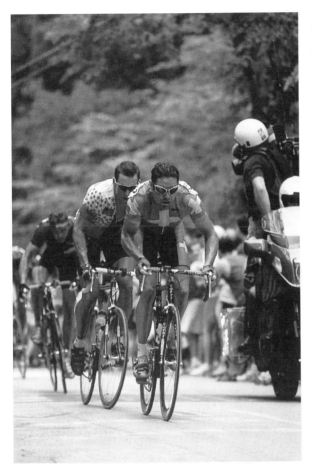

Fig. 6.14 Atlanta 1996: road race. Richard Pascal (SUI), first; Sciandri Maximilian (GBR), second, adjusting tactics because of heat and humidity. © Allsport / Mike Powell.

Short efforts are not likely to be hindered by heat and humidity. Events longer than 5 min will be raced at lower intensity.

Altitude and hypoxia

As one ascends, there is less barometric pressure, and less oxygen in the blood. This condition is called hypoxia. At sea level, the average barometric pressure is 760 mmHg. At 3000 m the barometer reads 510 mmHg. The percentage of oxygen in the air (about 21%), does not change, but the density of oxygen does. Only two-thirds of sea-level oxygen is present.

Details concerning physiological adaptations and the use of altitude as a training aid are not discussed here.

Altitude illnesses

Altitude sickness. Many who travel to altitude experience side-effects. Most people adapt to altitude more quickly when they have travelled to high altitudes frequently in the past. Side-effects are not predictable. Some individuals may have problems on some occasions and not on others. Problems occur in proportion to the change in altitude. Those living at sea level have more problems when travelling to 2500 m than those living at 1000 m. Changes in altitude of less than 1000 m do not present much difficulty.

At 2500 m and above, headache, drowsiness, mental fatigue, dizziness, nausea, vomiting, insomnia, dimness of vision (especially colour vision) and euphoria may occur. Judgement and memory are ordinarily normal to 3000 m. At 3500 m, reaction times, handwriting and psychology test scores may be 20% below normal. Pulmonary oedema, convulsions and coma can occur above 7000 m.

Short-term acclimatization is usually complete by 2 weeks. Many riders have a bad day between the second and fifth days at altitude.

Reduced aerobic capacity. At 1500 m, $V_{O_{2max}}$, or the body's maximum ability to use oxygen, is reduced by about 5%. At 2000 m it is reduced by about 7.5%. Thinking about training at Pikes Peak or riding up Mount Evans (about 4000 m) in Colorado? There will be about a 25% reduction in V_{O_2}.

The reduced amount of oxygen means that less work can be performed. Cycling time-trial records are often accomplished at altitude because the reduced ability to work is more than compensated for by reduced air resistance. But athletes in sports with less aerodynamic benefit, such as running, do worse in aerobic events at altitude.

Even when adapted, one cannot sustain the same levels of aerobic work as at sea level. For a given work load, heart rate may be higher. Since one cannot work as hard at altitude, the threshold working heart rate may be lower. For a given speed on the level, heart rate may be lower.

Acid–base balance. There is a change in the acid–base balance in the body. Breathing fast means that carbon dioxide levels in the blood fall. This changes the

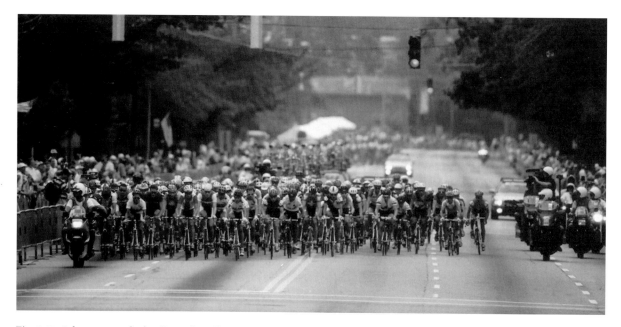

Fig. 6.15 Atlanta 1996: the leading riders all must deal with heat and humidity. © Allsport / Stu Forster.

blood pH and results in the kidneys losing bicarbonate. This may mean that the body is less able to buffer lactic acid.

Dehydration and sunburn. The air at altitude is usually very dry. Extra fluids may be lost due to increased breathing. Since fluid losses are greater, it is easier to become dehydrated. Sun intensity is also higher. Be sure to drink plenty of fluids, and protect skin and lips with sunscreens.

Acclimatization

If one is travelling to an important event and has the time, one strategy is to arrive 3 weeks early. Ride at an easy pace for the first few days, train hard the second week and taper the third. Another strategy is to arrive at the last possible moment and hope for the best.

Many races are over a range of altitudes. If you do not have the time to acclimatize, it may be helpful to rest and sleep at lower elevations when not racing.

Fatigue and overtraining

For both athletes and non-athletes alike, fatigue is one of the most common reasons why patients see physicians. The differential diagnosis is large and it is not always possible to arrive at a diagnosis.

Many athletic trainers and coaches often assume that overtraining is the explanation for fatigue in their athletes. Our understanding of overtraining is in its infancy. There are, as yet, no sensitive and specific markers for overtraining. Diagnosis is often uncertain. Frequently, other factors cause fatigue or confound the diagnosis. What follows is some of the limited information we currently have about these problems.

Fatigue

Riders may find themselves tired and wonder why. Fatigue probably falls into one of these categories:
1 stress or emotional turmoil;
2 inadequate sleep;
3 too rapid weight loss;
4 inadequate nutrition;
5 medical problems, including depression;
6 overtraining or burnout.

Stress

Stress is one of the most common reasons why athletes and non-athletes are tired. Most people think of stress as bad events in their lives. Actually, stress is change.

Good changes and bad changes are stressful. Buying a new bicycle and figuring out all the components to put on it and being excited about it may be good, but increased anxiety may cause you sleep loss and exhaustion just in planning – never mind riding – a new bike. Marriages, separations, deaths in the family, job changes, moving, new purchases and accidents are some of the big stresses in our lives. Too many in a year cause most of us to become tired, perhaps as a psychological way of avoiding these stressful situations.

Consider the important people and things in life: family and friends, job and money. Have your circumstances changed recently? If so, stress may contribute to fatigue.

Inadequate sleep

Sleep loss is an understandable cause of fatigue. Inadequate sleep is often related to stresses, discussed above. By going to sleep at a regular hour and rising at a regular hour you set the pattern for good sleep habits. Quiet activity 15 min before sleep – reading a book or listening to soft music – may also help the cyclist to sleep better.

Too rapid weight loss

Many athletes rightly try to lose weight to improve their performance. Weight loss of more than 0.5–1 kg weekly, though, often results in fatigue and worsens performance.

Inadequate nutrition

The body needs calories, nutrients and fluids to work properly. If you ride for more than a couple of hours and become tired, the problem may be simply that you need to eat and drink more. Chronic glycogen depletion is a common cause of fatigue.

Medical causes

If fatigue lasts for more than a month or two, a medical check-up may be wise. Some causes include anaemia, diabetes, low thyroid levels and other organ disease of almost any kind, infectious diseases and depression.

Depression is an extremely common medical illness, characterized by fatigue and irritability. Although emotional lows or sadness may be present, many people with medical depression do not report these feelings. Interrupted sleep, change in sex drive, pain, lack of enjoyment, change in bowel habits, difficulty concentrating and worthless feelings characterize depression. These symptoms often overlap with those of overtraining, which is discussed below. Depression is effectively treated with antidepressant medication.

Chronic fatigue syndrome is a poorly understood medical condition. No consistent physical findings, laboratory tests, causes or treatments exist. As is the case with other medical problems that remain poorly defined, personal testimonial and anecdotal reports, often related with considerable conviction, cloud scientific evidence. At one time the Epstein–Barr virus was thought to be related to this problem. Current evidence dismisses this possibility. Some patients' symptoms may be improved by the simple addition of salt to their diets. It is clear that depression is often present.

Overtraining

Overtraining includes exercise fatigue, burnout, apathy, lethargy or staleness in otherwise healthy athletes. Many people think of overtraining as a physical condition, and burnout as a psychological or emotional one. They are intertwined, since most psychological states have a physical, biochemical, metabolic and/or neurohormonal basis.

Overtraining is an imbalance of training and recovery, exercise and exercise capacity. The training effect is the body's response to work load stress. If stress is too great, the body cannot respond and adapt and overtraining may result. (*Overloading* is a building or anabolic adaptation to work load stress. *Overtraining* is a breakdown or catabolic response. *Overuse* is musculoskeletal overtraining.)

Maximizing human performance requires great volumes of intense training without overtraining. Some say: 'Put the finger near the fire to know that it is hot, but do not burn it!' Overtraining symptoms include:

1 poor, non-restorative sleep;
2 mood disturbances, including anxiety, irritability, loss of enjoyment and sadness;

3 poor performance with the same or increased training;

4 vague or undefined physical complaints.

A combination of training and non-training stresses affect athletes. *Training stresses* include:

1 too much volume;

2 too much intensity;

3 too little recovery.

Common situations that result in training stress include:

1 excess competition;

2 attempts to follow a training plan when injured or ill;

3 inappropriate increased training in an attempt to make up for rest related to injury or illness;

4 inappropriate increased training in an attempt to make up for poor competition performance.

Non-training stresses include:

1 excessive work, school or family responsibilities;

2 interpersonal conflict with coworkers or bosses, friends or family;

3 drug problems;

4 housing problems;

5 money problems;

6 legal problems;

7 illness or injury in self or others;

8 insufficient sleep;

9 poor diet.

Short- and long-term overtraining

Short-term overtraining may be related to local muscle factors, including depletion of glycogen or muscle injury. Long-term overtraining involves, in addition, neurohormonal factors in the nervous system, including the brain and endocrine glands.

Short-term overtraining, also called overreaching or isolated peripheral overtraining, is characterized by:

1 taking a few days to 2 weeks to develop;

2 exercise fatigue;

3 reduction of submaximal performance capacity;

4 reduction of maximum performance capacity;

5 short-term competitive incompetence;

6 recovery achieved within days;

7 favourable prognosis.

Long-term overtraining, also called overtraining syndrome, staleness or combination peripheral and central overtraining, is characterized by:

1 taking weeks to months to develop;

2 exercise and non-exercise fatigue;

3 reduction of submaximal performance capacity;

4 reduction of maximum performance capacity;

5 mood disturbance;

6 muscle soreness or stiffness;

7 long-term competitive incompetence;

8 recovery requiring weeks to months;

9 uncertain prognosis.

Diagnosis

Clinical symptoms, athletic performance and medical tests point to the diagnosis. No test is foolproof or perfect; for some symptoms and tests, other medical problems give similar profiles. In self-monitoring, the best-known markers to watch for are:

1 morning weight down more than 3%;

2 hours of sleep down more than 10%;

3 resting heart rate increased more than 10%;

4 mood changes, including fatigue, loss of enthusiasm and depression.

Research has suggested that a number of changes occur with overtraining:

1 Maximum heart rate decreases.

2 Hormone changes:

(a) cortisol: resting and 8 a.m. blood levels increase; postexercise levels decrease;

(b) catecholamines (dopamine, adrenaline and noradrenaline) decrease in urine at night by more than 50%. They increase relatively more for the same intensity of exercise;

(c) testosterone blood levels decrease;

(d) insulin responsiveness decreases.

3 Blood chemistry changes: firstly, triglycerides, low-density and very-low-density lipoprotein lipids decrease, and secondly, maximum lactate and sub-maximum lactate decreases. Submaximum levels may (falsely) give the impression of improved performance. The ratio of blood lactate to perceived exertion decreases.

4 Neurotransmitters change: serotonin levels in the brain increase.

5 Immunoglobins and the immune system changes: immunoglobulin A in saliva decreases.

6 Muscle energy and water stores change in short-term overtraining syndrome:

(a) glycogen is depleted;

(b) intracellular stores of water are reduced.

Prevention

  1 Individualize training.
  2 Do not increase the frequency, duration or intensity too quickly.
  3 Allow for recovery. Plan and schedule rest days and longer rest cycles.
  4 A good endurance base is required before interval work.
  5 Sleep at least 8 h a night.
  6 Consider afternoon naps, rest or meditation.
  7 Review non-training stresses, and attempt to reduce or accommodate them.
  8 Avoid overcompensating for time missed from training.
  9 Avoid overcompensating for poor race performance.
10 Adjust goals.
11 Eat a nutritionally sound high-carbohydrate diet to help prevent glycogen depletion.
12 Hydrate.
13 Monitor morning pulse, weight loss and sleep patterns for self-diagnosis of overtraining.

Treatment

Since overtraining is the result of an imbalance between training and recovery, treatment is directed at reducing training load or increasing recovery.

Symptoms, athletic performance and medical tests are often the same or overlap considerably in overtraining and medical depression. Some think that overtraining is a cause of medical depression. Medical depression also lessens the ability to train. Preliminary scientific investigation suggests that antidepressant medication may help athletes train harder, treat overtraining syndrome and improve performance.

Exercise and immunity

The effects of aerobic exercise in general, and of bicycling in particular, on the immune system are uncertain. The study of the immune system is in its infancy. Preliminary information suggests that the acute or short-term effects of exercise are to lower, or worsen, the immune system. Chronic (long-term) regular exercise may help the immune system.

The immune system appears to decline with age. Some of this decline may be offset by a programme of lifelong regular aerobic exercise.

General treatment options

The following is a brief review of standard treatment options.

RICE – rest, ice, compression and elevation

This classic initial treatment of injuries comprises four parts.

Rest

Rest helps almost all injuries. The degree of rest needed depends on the injury. For many injuries, modified rest is all that is necessary – a reduction in mileage, a lessening of hill work or big-gear riding. A minimal ankle twist may require only caution for a day or two to avoid reinjury. A mild ankle sprain may require avoiding sports for a couple of days.

A severe ankle sprain may require casting. This is really just a method of enforced rest for a part of the body. Sometimes, as with a broken bone, complete rest may be required. Partial casts and splints represent less extreme forms of enforced rest.

In general, if activity makes the injury more painful, avoid the activity.

Ice

The application of local cold reduces injury-induced pain, inflammation and swelling. Apply ice for no more than 15 min at a time every hour. Direct ice to the skin can cause skin freezing and damage. Wrap ice in a cloth to prevent direct contact with the skin.

Ice is the key, but it is not necessarily used. Some prefer a package of frozen vegetables. Frozen peas, for example, conform easily to the surface of the damaged body part and can be used repeatedly. (But do not eat those peas subsequently!) Instant ice – commercial preparations that chill when internal physical partitions are broken, allowing chemicals to contact and react with one another – are convenient, expensive and relatively short-lived in action.

Compression

Compressing the injured area prevents fluid from entering and reduces swelling. Compression also provides a modest form of enforced rest.

Avoid compressing so tightly that the circulation is impaired. Compression applied closer to the heart should not be as strong as that applied further away. Numbness, tingling, pale or bluish skin may result from compression that is too tight.

Compression applied before swelling has formed is usually better than that applied after swelling is already present. To be effective, compression must be selective. In ankle injury, for example, most injuries occur in depressions. Padding under the wrap at these depressions improves the effectiveness of compression.

There are many different products on the market for compression use. In an ankle injury, an elastic wrap provides modest compression but not much support. Specialty products, such as an ankle air-cast support, provide significantly more effective compression and support.

Elevation

Raising the injured part to the level of the heart reduces local swelling. For example, injuries to the arm are often elevated using a sling. Leg injuries are elevated by sitting and raising the leg, for example, on another chair.

Non-steroidal anti-inflammatory drugs

NSAIDs are medicines against inflammation. They also ease pain. Sometimes one works well where others do not. A few are available over-the-counter without a prescription, for example, in the USA, aspirin, ibuprofen (Advil) and naproxen (Aleve). The rest are on prescription only.

Many medical problems are due to inflammation. Inflammation is a reaction of the body when it attempts to heal itself from injury or infection. Sometimes the body fights too hard, and excessive inflammation leads to pain, discomfort or disability.

Dosing

Aspirin and ibuprofen only last for a few hours, and so often require many daily doses to be helpful. Several medicines in the group need to be taken only once or twice a day. Manufacturers are formulating more of these products to last longer. In general, medications

that require more frequent dosing have a faster onset of action.

In general these medicines are used in one of three ways:
1 as-needed dosing: medicine is taken with pain;
2 anticipatory dosing: medicine is taken in anticipation of pain, to prevent pain and inflammation;
3 regular dosing: medicine is taken regularly for a period of days to break a pain cycle, or to reduce inflammation sufficiently to improve the condition.

Side-effects

A common problem with this class of medicines is an upset GI tract. Table 6.6 lists the relative degree of GI upset caused by these medicines. There is some evidence that anti-inflammatory drugs impede fracture healing. Some orthopaedic surgeons avoid their use for pain control when there is a fracture.

Physical therapy

Physical therapy provides a variety of healing methods for acute and chronic conditions. The conditions may result from overuse, degeneration, injury or surgery. The use of these methods is not restricted to physical therapists. Physicians, athletic trainers, osteopaths and chiropractors may all have education and experience in using all or some of these methods.

Physical therapy involves not only the treatment itself, but the education and instruction of patients. It often provides important psychological support for patients. It may consist of the following types of programmes:
1 Range-of-motion exercises. These increase the range of motion of joints. Passive range-of-motion exercises are joint motions performed without muscle force, either by the patient or by another person. These exercises are sometimes performed with the assistance of gravity or traction as the moving force. Active range-of-motion exercises are joint motions performed with muscular force. The patient actively uses muscular force to increase the range of motion.
2 Stretching. This increases the length of ligaments or tendons. Stretching is helpful in preventing and treating overuse injuries. Many overuse injuries are the result of too much stress or tension on a tendon.

Table 6.6 Non-steroidal anti-inflammatory drugs: common agents, doses and side-effects.

Class and agent	Doses per day	Gastrointestinal side-effects
Fenamotos		
Meclofenamate sodium (Meclomen)	4	3
Mefenamic acid (Ponstel)	4	1
Indoles		
Indomethacin (Indocin)	2–3	4
Indomethacin (Indocin SR)	1	4
Sulindac (Clinoril)	2	1
Tolmetin sodium (Tolectin)	3–4	3
Napthykanone		
Nabumetone (Relafen)	2	2
Oxicam		
Piroxicam (Feldene)	1	3
Phenylacetic acid		
Diclofenac sodium (Voltaren)	4	2
Propionic acids		
Fenoprofen calcium (Nalfon)	3–4	2
Flurbiprofen (Ansaid)	3–4	2
Ibuprofen (Advil, Motrin)	3–4	2
Ketoprofen (Orudis)	3–4	2
Naproxen (Naprosyn)	2	2
Naproxen sodium (Naprelan, Aleve, Anaprox)	1–2	2
Oxaprosin (Daypro)	1	1
Pyranocarboxylic acid		
Etodolac (Lodine)	3	1
Pyrazoles		
Phenylbutazone (Azoid, Butazolidin)	4	4
Pyrrolopyrrole		
Ketorolac tromethamine (Toradol)	4	3
Salicylates		
Acetylsalicylic acid (Aspirin)	4	4
Diflunisal (Dolobid)	2	1

Doses range from 1 to 4 daily. Gastrointestinal upset ranges from 1 (minimal) to 4 (most).

Stretching the muscles and tendons allows them to absorb more strain without discomfort. Be cautious about stretching when injured. Use stretching primarily to prevent reinjury. For some specific overuse injuries, particular stretches are helpful (see under relevant sections, above).

3 Strengthening programmes. These strengthen specific muscles. Strengthening exercises may help to rehabilitate or cure many problems. Be cautious about strength training with an injury and use it primarily to prevent reinjury. It is important to understand what the exercise is meant to accomplish and to perform it correctly. For example, leg extension performed only for the last 20° of extension – so called short-arc or terminal extension exercises – help many knee problems. Full-extension exercises worsen many knee problems.

4 Massage. Massage provides pain relief and helps muscular relaxation. There is little controlled, scientific understanding about how this works.

5 Whirlpool baths. These provide a massage-type effect. Whirlpool is also helpful for the gentle removal of scabs or scab-like material from abrasions, burns or other wounds.

6 Cold. This prevents local swelling or provides pain relief. It is thought to decrease the local circulation. Cold is generally applied for the first 48 h after an injury or while swelling is present. Cold is discussed in greater detail on p. 113.

7 Heat. Heat increases the local circulation which is thought to speed the healing process. It is generally applied after injuries, when swelling has gone down. Heat may be local and applied directly, such as with heating pads, hot-water bottles and hot baths. It may be local and applied indirectly, such as with infrared light. Heat may be deep, such as that provided by diathermy and ultrasound. Be careful that you do not burn the skin: burns from heating pads are common. Heat should not cause significant pain or redness when applied. Do not use heat or cold on areas of the skin that are numb or suffer from decreased circulation. It is easy to freeze or burn skin that does not sense temperature properly.

8 Ultrasound. Sound waves penetrate the tissues, causing local heat. It may also provide benefit by vibrating the tissues, but this is uncertain.

9 Electrotherapy. Electrical currents applied to the skin may help chronic pain. Electrotherapy includes the *transcutaneous electrical nerve stimulation (TENS)* unit.

10 Manipulation. This method is unpopular with the US medical profession because of its association with chiropractic. Studies support its effectiveness for certain specific problems, including back pain.

Other treatment options

Orthotics

These shoe inserts help support the foot and direct weight and energy forces. Orthotics may provide support, cant (angle) the foot, or provide a space or shim to help correct a small leg-length discrepancy. They are used for a variety of foot, ankle, knee, hip, back and other biomechanical problems. Cycling orthotics are longer than running orthotics: they should support the metatarsal heads.

Orthotics may be modest over-the-counter products used interchangeably by different individuals and in different sports, or sport-specific customized products costing hundreds of dollars.

They may help those in whom anatomical variation is otherwise difficult to correct by adjusting the bicycle. Orthotics may be helpful in realigning the structures of the leg. They tend to be most useful for problems closer to the foot and less useful for such problems as back and neck ache.

Those who walk with an abnormal pressure pattern (Fig. 6.16) are most likely to be helped with orthotics. If chronic foot, knee, hip or leg pain or problems exist, and foot patterns are abnormal, it is possible that an orthotic may help.

If foot patterns are abnormal and no problems exist, there is no reason to use orthotics. For those who have needed orthotics, studies have shown no difference in power when cycling with orthotics. Orthotics may help pain or other medical problems, but do not otherwise improve performance.

Shims

Leg-length discrepancy is usually corrected by the use of a shim placed between the cleat and shoe. Approximately one-third to one-half of the discrepancy is corrected. The bicycle is adjusted to fit the longer leg.

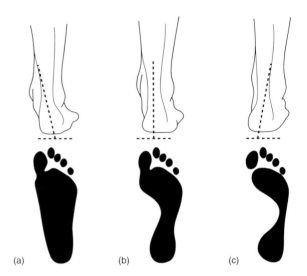

Fig. 6.16 Foot patterns. (a) Pronation abnormal pattern; (b) normal pattern; and (c) supination abnormal pattern.

Wedges

These canted shims may help overcome pronation or supination stress.

Muscle relaxants

This is a group of popular medicines. Some pharmacologists dispute their specificity. My feeling is that they relax the brain as much as the muscles. Most people have a natural tendency towards depression when injured. I believe muscle relaxants often increase an individual's depression. I do not think they usually have significant value in the treatment of injuries.

Pain medicine

Analgesia may be needed for sudden injuries. A combination pill containing paracetamol (acetaminophen: Tylenol) and codeine is the most widely prescribed pain medicine. This is stronger than over-the-counter medicine.

Codeine is a narcotic. Use what is needed for pain control, but not more. If aspirin, ibuprofen (Advil) or paracetamol is sufficient, there is no need to suffer the narcotic side-effects of constipation and mental dullness.

If NSAIDs are used for inflammation as well as for pain control, one may wish to continue their use even after pain has diminished.

Cortisone

Cortisone is a natural body hormone, but its products have also been synthesized as drugs with massive potencies. They are available as oral, topical and injectable medications. Local injections allow a strong anti-inflammatory to be placed at the inflamed structure. They are powerful methods of relieving inflammation, but have some serious side-effects. For example, they can cause weakness and rupture of a tendon. For this reason, they are inappropriate for Achilles and patellar tendons.

Surgery

This is the most invasive tool to solve problems. Sometimes it is the first choice in helping a broken bone or other serious injury. For overuse injuries, surgery is most often a last resort.

Further reading

Baker, A. (1998) *Bicycling Medicine*. Simon & Schuster, New York.

Bartok-Oslon, C.J. & Keith, R.E. (1996) Prevalence of eating disorder symptoms in female collegiate college cyclists. *Medicine and Science in Sports and Exercise* **28** (Suppl.), May.

Birnbaum, J.S. (1986) *The Musculoskeletal Manual*. Grune & Stratton, Orlando, FL.

Brechtel, L.M. & Braumann, K.M. (1996) Non-responding of the sympatho-adrenal system – a diagnostic sign for the overtraining syndrome. *Medicine and Science in Sports and Exercise* **28** (Suppl.), May.

Broker, J.P. & Gregor, R.J. (1990) A dual piezoelectric element force pedal for kinetic analysis of cycling. *International Journal of Sports Biomechanics* **6**, 394–403.

Broker, J.P. & Gregor, R.J. (1996) Cycling biomechanics. In: *High-tech Cycling* (ed E.R. Burke), pp. 145–66, Human Kinetics, Champaign, IL.

Burke, R.E. & Edgerton, V.R. (1975) Motor unit properties and selective involvement in humans. In: *Exercise and Sport Science Review* (eds J.H. Wilmore & J.F. Keogh) Academic Press, New York.

Danh, K., Mai, L., Poland, J. & Jenkins, C. (1991) Frictional resistance in bicycle wheel bearings. *Cycling Science* **3**(3–4), 44–50.

Francis, P.R. (1986) Injury prevention for cyclists: A biomechanical approach. In: *Science of Cycling* (ed E.R. Burke), pp. 145–84, Human Kinetics, Champaign, IL.

Francis, P.R. (1988) Pathomechanics of the lower extremity in cycling. In: *Medical and Scientific Aspects of Cycling* (eds E.R. Burke & M.M. Newsome), pp. 3–16, Human Kinetics, Champaign, IL.

Garrick, J. & Webb, D. (1990) *Sports Injuries, Diagnosis and Management*. Saunders, Philadelphia.

Gisolfi, C., Maughn, R. & Schiller, L. (1993) Intestinal fluid absorption in exercise and disease. *Sport Science Exchange* **11**. http://www.gssiweb.com.

Gisolfi, C.V., Rohlf, D.P., Navarude, S.N. *et al.* (1988) Effects of wearing a helmet on thermal balance while cycling in the heat. *Physician Sports Medicine* **16**, 139.

Gregor, R.J. & Fowler, E. (1996) Biomechanics of Cycling. In: *Athletic Injuries and Rehabilitation* (eds J.J. Zachazewski,

D.J. MaGee & W.S. Quillan), pp. 367–88, W.B. Saunders Co, Philadelphia, PA.

Gregor, R.J., Cavanagh, R.R. & La Fortune, M. (1985) Knee flexor moments during propulsion in cycling: a creative solution to Lombard's paradox. *Journal of Biomechanics* **18**, 307–16.

Gulledge, T.P. & Hackney, A.C. (1996) Reproducibility of low resting testosterone levels in endurance trained men. *Medicine and Science in Sports and Exercise* **28** (Suppl.), May.

Guyton, A. (1971) *Textbook of Medical Physiology*. Saunders, Philadelphia.

Hannaford, D.R., Moran, G.T. & Hlavac, H.F. (1986) Video analysis and treatment of overuse knee injury in cycling: A limited clinical study. *Clinics in Podiatric Medicine and Surgery* **3**, 671–78.

Hyatt, J.P. & Clarkson, P.M. (1996) Exercise-induced muscle damage in subjects with different levels of ingested estrogen. *Medicine and Science in Sports and Exercise* **28** (Suppl.), May.

Kyle, C.R. (1988) How friction slows a bike. *Bicycling* **June**, 180–85.

Kyle, C.R. (1995) Bicycle aerodynamics. In: *Human Powered Vehicles* (eds A.V. Abbott & D.G. Wilson), pp. 141–55, Human Kinetics, Champaign, IL.

Kyle, C.R. (1996) Selecting cycling equipment. In: *High-tech Cycling* (ed E.R. Burke), pp. 1–43, Human Kinetics, Champaign, IL.

Lamb, D.R. (1984) *Physiology of Exercise – Responses and Adaptations*. Macmillan, New York.

Lieber, R.L. (1992) *Skeletal Muscle Structure and Function: Implications for Rehabilitation and Sports Medicine*. Williams & Wilkins, Baltimore, MD, USA.

Manjra, S., Schwellnus, M.P. & Noakes, T.D. (1996) Risk factors for exercise associated muscle cramping. *Medicine and Science in Sports and Exercise* **28** (Suppl.), May.

Maughen, R. & Rehrer, N. (1993) Gastric emptying during exercise. *Sports Science Exchange* **46**. http://www.gssiweb.com.

McArdle, W., Katch, F. & Katch, V. (1994) *Exercise Physiology*. Lea & Feibiger, Philadelphia.

McCoy, R.W. (1989) *The effect of varying seat position on knee loads during cycling*. Unpublished doctoral dissertation, University of Southern California, Department of Exercise Science.

Mellion, M.B. & Burke, E. (1994) *Clinics in Sports Medicine, Bicycling Injuries*. Saunders, Philadelphia.

Millar, A.L., Blakely, J. & Blakely, M. (1999) The effects of massage on delayed onset muscle soreness, force production and physiological parameters. *Medicine and Science in Sports and Exercise* **28** (Suppl.), May.

Peronnet, F., Bouissou, P., Perrault, H. & Ricci, J. (1992) Three-dimensional knee loading during seated cycling. *Journal of Biomechanics* **25**, 1195–207.

Ryan, M.M. & Gregor, R.J. (1992) EMG profiles of lower extremity muscles during cycling at constant workload and cadence. *Journal of Electromyography and Kinesiology* **2**, 69–80.

Sanderson, D.J. (1990) The biomechanics of cycling shoes. *Cycling Science* **Sept.**, 27–30.

Sherman, W. (1990) Exercise and type I diabetes. *Sports Science Exchange* **25**. http://www.gssiweb.com.

Sherman, W. (1992) Exercise and type II diabetes. *Sports Science Exchange* **37**. http://www.gssiweb.com.

Terrados, N., Fernandez, B., Perez Landaluce, J. & Rodriguez, M. (1996) Hormonal changes during a professional cycling road race. *Medicine and Science in Sports and Exercise* **28** (Suppl.), May.

Thompson, H.S., Hyatt, J.P. & Clarkson, P.M. (1996) Exercise-induced muscle damage in subjects with different levels of ingested oestrogen. *Medicine & Science in Sports and Exercise*, Suppl. **28**, 5th May.

Walmsley, B. & Proske, U. (1981) Comparison of stiffness of soleus and medical gastrocnemius muscles in cats. *Journal of Neurophysiology* **46**, 250–59.

Weiss, B.D. (1994) Bicycle-related head injuries. In: *Clinics in Sports Medicine* (eds M.B. Mellior & E.R. Burke). Saunders, Philadelphia.

Wheeler, J.B. (1993) Applied MZ moment patterns at the shoe/pedal interface: A biomechanical analysis of clip-less pedals, float features, and their implications for overuse knee injuries during cycling. Unpubhlished master's thesis, University of California, Los Angeles.

Wheeler, J.B., Gregor, R.J. & Broker, J.P. (1995) The effect of clipless float designs on shoe/pedal interface kinetics: implications for overuse knee injuries during cycling. *Journal of Applied Biomechanics* **11**, 119–41.

Williams, M.H., Kreidis, R.B. & Branch, B.J. (1999) *Creatine: The Power Supplement*. Human Kinetics Publications, Champaign DL.

Wilson, J.D. & Braunwald, E. (1991) *Harrison's Textbook of Internal Medicine*. McGraw Hill, New York.

Index

Please note: page numbers in *italic* refer to figures and those in **bold** refer to tables.